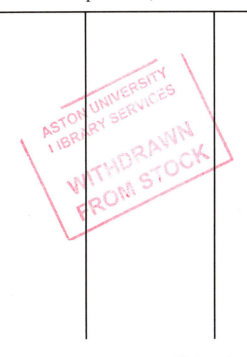

Intelligent Software for Product Formulation

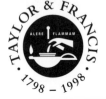

Intelligent Software for Product Formulation

RAYMOND C. ROWE, BPharm, PhD, DSc, FRPharmS, CChem, FRSC, CPhys, MInstP

RONALD J. ROBERTS, BSc, PhD

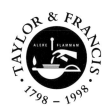

UK Taylor & Francis Ltd, 1 Gunpowder Square, London EC4A 3DE
USA Taylor & Francis Inc., 1900 Frost Road, Suite 101, Bristol, PA 19007–1598

British Library Cataloguing in Publication Data
A catalogue record for this book is available from the British Library
ISBN 0-7484-0732-4 (cased)

Library of Congress Cataloging Publication Data are available

Cover design by Jim Wilkie

Typeset in Times 10/12pt by Graphicraft Typesetters Ltd, Hong Kong

Printed in Great Britain by T.J. International Ltd, Padstow, UK

'It is unworthy for men of excellence to labour like slaves over tasks that could be safely relegated to machines'

Liebnitz (1646–1716)

but

'If you turn to a computer to solve a problem you do not understand, all you're doing is transferring your lack of understanding to a technology you do not understand'

Angell (1991)

Contents

Foreword

With the exception of pressurised metered dose inhalers, all common forms of a medicine existed before the beginning of this century. They evolved empirically in the hands of chemists only dimly aware of how product efficacy, stability and elegance were achieved. Their legacy is a range of medicines which combine chemical and physical characteristics in a most complex manner. The modern pharmaceutical scientist (and the authors are two of the most eminent) may try to unravel the basic principles of a formulation but only partial elucidation is likely. A successful outcome will inevitably involve a formulation expert. His judgements will be subjective based on a product's consistency, appearance and a range of empirical tests, such as snapping a tablet between the fingers. The disadvantages of this are obvious. Skills are slowly acquired and a crucial resource is lost with the loss of personnel. Since assessments are subjective, they cannot be transferred up and down an organisational hierarchy, leaving junior staff without a secure learning process and managers impotent to influence a technical outcome. This situation is a dynamic one in which the criteria of product assessment are becoming more stringent with the introduction into a specification of new clauses defining particle size distribution, bioburden, dissolution rate, rheometry, more searching impurity patterns and so on.

Meeting both old and new criteria will be facilitated if the total experimental experience of a group of technologists could be brought to bear rather than the uncertain extension of an empirical comprehension to achieve refined objectives. Such a process can be carried out by intelligent software systems.

Whether pursuing fundamental science or their expert systems, the authors have always scrutinised technologies from other industries to achieve their pharmaceutical objectives. They quote the oil industry where oxidation inhibitors, friction modifiers, viscosity modifiers, detergents and many other ingredients are added to a base to make up a modern lubricating oil. Interaction between components is complex, defying rigorous analysis and creating dependence on experienced formulators and expensive engine tests. The parallel with pharmaceutical formulation is almost exact, differing only in the pace of development. Other industries pose the same problem, always characterised by technology which outruns its scientific base.

A common thread links all formulators and the authors demonstrate that the experience gained by the empiricist in these diverse industrial situations can itself be 'formulated' in a way which permits interrogation by any intelligent technologist. Provided the knowledge base is skilfully constructed, a highly efficient, reproducible and durable expert system can be used to tap the enormous but diffuse body of knowledge often painfully acquired by companies struggling with the vagaries of conventional formulation over many years. However, the contribution of such systems to modern formulation practice is not properly exploited. There are many reasons for this. There is the frank sceptic who does not believe that artificial intelligence can be adequately developed to solve a formulator's problems. At the other end of the spectrum, there is a willing technologist unable to harness expert systems and neural networks. This text seeks to disarm the former and encourage and assist the latter. It does so in clear stages. It first describes the tools and then the interaction between experts and the knowledge engineer. Rather than deal in depth with artificial intelligence, it details the construction and use of a product formulation expert system as an exemplar. Readers wishing to go further are helped by extensive references. Neural networks, genetic algorithms and fuzzy logic are described at a level which illustrates their potential usefulness to the formulator. The reader is now equipped to consider applications and may well be surprised at the level of technological diversity. Whilst the text reflects the authors' innovations in pharmaceuticals, examples range from textile finishing to Szechwan cooking.

Throughout, the text reflects the great enthusiasm of the authors for the contribution artificial intelligence can make to their work. However, no doubt mindful of the sceptics frequently encountered, they carefully balance costs and benefits objectively whether they are discussing the technical challenge, improved quality, savings in cost or accommodation of skill shortages. In so doing, they identify the situations in which intelligent software is likely to give greatest advantage. The presentation is such that on the one hand it will equip a technical manager to evaluate critically the broad contribution intelligent software might make. On the other, it will enable a formulator to identify how the technology might be applied to a specific activity. By meeting the needs of both, the authors will ensure that formulation will become quicker and the outcome more certain.

D. Ganderton, OBE

Preface

The introduction of a continuous stream of new and improved products is essential for a company to maintain its competitive advantage. The process of formulating these products, whether they be pharmaceuticals, agrochemicals, specialty chemicals or any one of a number of others from industries where product formulation occurs, is a highly specialised task requiring specific domain knowledge and often years of experience. Formulators are therefore a scarce resource and of high intrinsic value to their organisations. Intelligent software tools derived from research into artificial intelligence can assist the efficient formulation of products increasing productivity, consistency and quality.

We were first introduced to a subset of intelligent software, viz. expert systems, some ten years ago when, as members of the Physical Sciences Group in the Pharmaceutical Department of ICI Pharmaceuticals UK (now Zeneca Pharmaceuticals) in conjunction with knowledge engineers from ICI Corporate Management Services UK and consultants from Logica UK Ltd, we began working on the development of an expert system for formulating tablets. The success of this project combined with the subsequent development of other expert systems and the implementation of other intelligent software tools, viz. neural networks and genetic algorithms, has convinced us of the real benefit that can accrue from applying this technology.

The aim of this book is primarily to demonstrate the applicability of expert systems, neural networks, genetic algorithms and other intelligent software in product formulation. It is not meant to be a textbook on artificial intelligence. There are a plethora of these available and many are mentioned in the references to each chapter. Rather it is meant to be a guide to provide readers with sufficient background of the technology to be able to identify opportunities and, hopefully, to initiate projects.

Many of the applications included in this book are taken from the pharmaceutical industry. This is not only because we personally have first hand knowledge of this domain but also because there are several well documented pharmaceutical applications in the open literature. These applications are counterbalanced as much as possible by others in fields ranging from alloys to textiles to provide the broadest possible perspective. We have also included typical examples of both formulation and fault diagnosis expert systems in two appendices to illustrate the operation of such systems.

This book has been written in a style which we hope will be acceptable to:

1 Practising product formulators who wish to learn more about this exciting technology.

2 Managers of product development laboratories who wish to find out more about the applications of intelligent software and the impact, benefits and issues surrounding their implementation.

3 Postgraduate or graduate students in chemistry and pharmacy who wish to obtain a background knowledge of the technology before starting a career in product development.

Included in this book are two chapters not written by ourselves. Both provide an overview of two commercial software packages specifically developed for product formulation. One is on PFES, a tool developed by Logica UK Ltd for the development of product formulation expert systems, the other is on CAD/Chem, a tool developed by AI Ware Inc. for modelling and optimising product formulations. The first is written by Paul Bentley, a Principal Consultant from Logica, the second by Elizabeth Colbourn, Managing Director of Oxford Materials Ltd which acts as distributor for AI Ware Inc. in the UK. We thank them both for their contributions.

In conclusion we wish to thank all our colleagues throughout Zeneca and ICI who have helped us in the successful implementation of intelligent software within the domain of product formulation.

R.C. Rowe
R.J. Roberts

1

Product Formulation and Artificial Intelligence

1.1 Product Innovation and Life Cycle

In a competitive environment the introduction of a continuous stream of new products is essential for the profitability and possible survival of a company. Casson (1983) stated: 'Long-run growth requires either a steady geographical expansion of the market area or a continuous innovation of new products. In the long run only product innovation can avoid the constraint imposed by the size of the world market for a given product.'

The idea that all products have a limited life and that demand will decline over time has been captured in the concept of the product life cycle (Figure 1.1). When a new product is first introduced on the market demand is low due to uncertainty. After this stage and assuming the new product is accepted in the marketplace there is a rapid growth as demand increases. However, such growth is likely to reach a ceiling as the product attains maturity and demand levels out. Eventually demand for the product will decrease leading ultimately to obsolescence. The time-scale for each stage will vary from one product to another with cycles ranging from the order of many years for successful products to very short times for unsuccessful products. The general perception is that product life cycles are, in general, shortening, implying an increasing pressure on companies to innovate on a regular basis.

Although such concepts are relevant to all manufactured products, they are particularly important in the area of formulated products where various ingredients are mixed/blended and processed to produce novel effects. In this case it is possible to play variations on the product life cycle theme and to define two strategies for maintaining or increasing sales volume. One way is to substitute an old product with a new product consisting either of a new active ingredient blended with other ingredients to produce a similar or enhanced effect (Figure 1.2a) or to extend the life cycle of the old product by producing new formulations, for example, at different concentrations, of different colour etc. of the old active ingredient or even by finding more uses for it (Figure 1.2b). Such strategies are used by many industries using formulation to produce marketable products (Table 1.1).

1

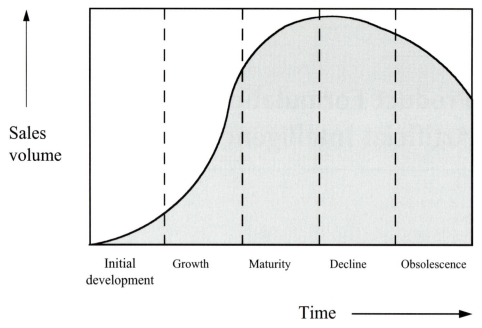

Figure 1.1   A generalised product life cycle

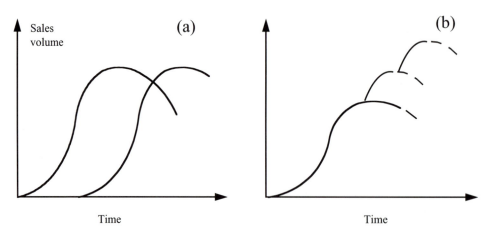

Figure 1.2   The effect on sales volume of two strategies: (a) substitution of a new product; (b) extension of life cycle

1.2   The Formulation Process

The process of formulation whether it be for pharmaceuticals, agrochemicals or specialty chemicals is generically the same, beginning with some form of product specification and ending with the generation of one or more formulations which meet the requirements. While the formulation consists of a list of ingredients and their proportions together with some processing variables where appropriate, the

Table 1.1 Examples of where product formulation is used

Industry	Tasks
Personal care	Sunscreens, skin creams, shampoos, bath gels
Pharmaceutical	Tablets, capsules, injections, creams
Cosmetics	Perfumes, make-up, nail varnish, lipstick
Foods/beverages	Confectionery, relishes, sauces, soft drinks
Paints/coatings	Primers, lacquers, varnishes, enamels
Adhesives	Pastes, glues
Lubricants	Oils, grease, mould releasing agents
Textiles	Dyestuffs, finishing agents, proofing agents
Agrochemicals	Emulsifiable concentrates, dispersible granules, sprays
Household chemicals	Polishes, cleaners, detergents
Photographic	Emulsions, developers, fixers
Miscellaneous	Alloys, refractories, inks, rubbers, plastics, composites, propellants, explosives, wall coverings

specification can vary considerably from one application to another. In some cases it may be very specific, expressed in terms of a performance level when subjected to a specific test, or quite general. It may also contain potentially conflicting performance criteria which the formulator may need to redefine in the light of experience. Figure 1.3 shows a typical formulation process broken down into its constituent tasks and sub-tasks (Bold, 1989).

In designing a formulation the formulator must take into account the properties of the active ingredient as well as possible chemical interactions between it and the other ingredients added to improve processibility and product properties since these may result in chemical instability. There may even be interactions between added ingredients leading to physical instability. Commercial factors as well as the policy of the industry towards ingredient usage are important influences, as are production factors in the intended markets. The formulator may also routinely access databases on previous formulations as well as make use of mathematical models. Figure 1.4 illustrates the information flow in this process. During the formulation process specific tests may need to be run to evaluate the properties of the proposed formulation. An analysis of unexpected results may lead to an adjustment of the ingredients and/or their levels.

The properties of the formulation are determined not only by the ratio in which the ingredients are combined but also by the processing conditions. Although relationships between ingredient levels, processing and product performance may be known anecdotally, rarely can they be precisely quantified. Models and simulations may be available but in many cases the formulation process has to be carried out in a design space that is multi-dimensional in nature and difficult to conceptualise.

This complexity can be clearly illustrated using the analogy of a jigsaw (Figure 1.5) where the total picture can only be seen when all the pieces are inserted in the correct orientation. However, even within the whole, subsets can be clearly defined, for example, product/properties/models or product/ingredients/costs. In all cases the formulator clearly has a pivotal role. It is not surprising, therefore, that formulation is a highly specialised task, requiring specific knowledge and often years of experience. This kind of expertise is not easily documented and hence senior

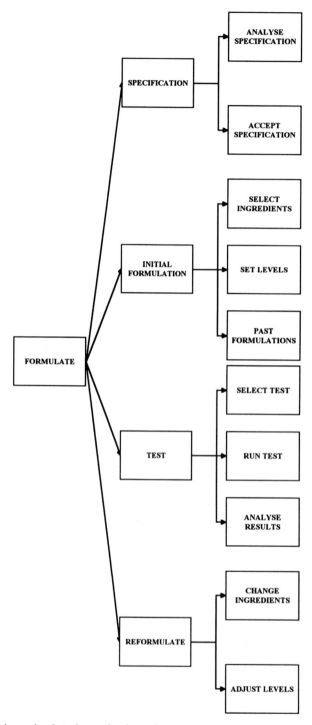

Figure 1.3 Tasks and sub-tasks in the formulation process

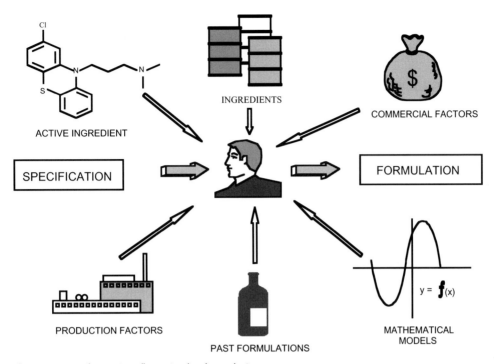

Figure 1.4 Information flows in the formulation process

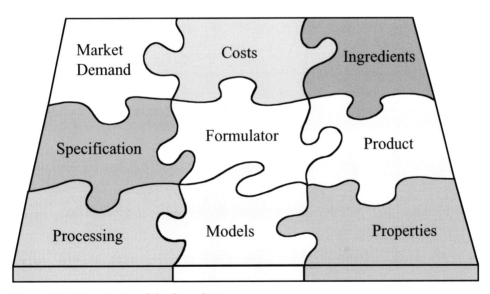

Figure 1.5 Complexity of the formulation process

formulators often spend considerable amounts of their time training new personnel. In addition, retirement or personnel moves can lead to a loss of irreplaceable commercial knowledge. Computer technology in the form of artificial intelligence (AI) provides an affordable means of capturing this knowledge and expertise in a documented form available to all.

1.3 Artificial Intelligence

Artificial intelligence is an interdisciplinary field which is often depicted as a tree with roots equating to the underlying disciplines (for example, linguistics, psychology, philosophy, biology, computer science and engineering) and the fruits of the canopy equating to the applications (for example, machine learning, problem solving, neural computing, computer vision, natural language processing, speech recognition, etc.; see Figure 1.6).

Because of this complexity no one definition of artificial intelligence has been universally accepted. However several exist:

> 'The capacity of a computer to perform tasks commonly associated with the higher intellectual processes characteristic of humans, such as the ability to reason, discover meanings, generalise, or learn from past experience' (*Encyclopaedia Britannica*, 1995).

> 'Artificial intelligence is the study of how to make computers do the things at which, at the moment, humans are better' (Rich, 1983).

> 'Artificial intelligence is an attempt to reproduce intelligent reasoning using machines' (Cartwright, 1993).

A definition more relevant to product formulation is that given by Turban (1995):

> 'Artificial intelligence is that part of computer science dealing with symbolic, non-algorithmic methods of problem solving'.

This definition focuses on three characteristics of importance in product formulation:

1   Problem solving – formulation has been described as a complex problem where the result is the best compromise available.

2   Symbolic processing – formulators do not solve problems by using sets of equations but by using symbols to represent the problem concepts and applying various strategies and rules to manipulate these concepts.

3   Non-algorithmic processing – formulators tend not to use an algorithmic approach (a well defined stepwise procedure guaranteed to reach a solution) to solving problems.

The potential value of artificial intelligence can be better understood by contrasting it with natural intelligence under various headings (Turban, 1995).

- Performance – natural intelligence is perishable due to personnel changes. Artificial intelligence is permanent as long as the computer systems remain unchanged.

- Ease of duplication/dissemination – natural intelligence in the form of expertise is difficult to transfer without a lengthy process of apprenticeship. Artificial intelligence in the form of a computer program can be easily duplicated and moved from one computer to another.

- Cost – artificial intelligence can be less expensive than natural intelligence. The cost of computing is decreasing daily while personnel costs are still increasing.

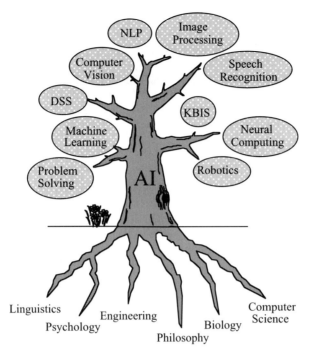

Figure 1.6 Artificial intelligence with disciplines (the tree roots) and applications (the tree fruits). DSS, decision support systems; KBIS, knowledge-based information systems; NLP, natural language processing

- Consistency – artificial intelligence, being a computer technology, is consistent compared with the unpredictability of human nature.
- Ease of documentation – decisions made by a computer can be easily traced and documented. Natural intelligence is difficult to document.
- Creativity – natural intelligence is creative whereas artificial intelligence is uninspired. The latter also requires direction.
- Focus – systems based on artificial intelligence are, by their very nature, focused. In contrast humans use a wide context of experience in problem solving.
- Sensory experience – humans are able to use sensory experience directly; systems based on artificial intelligence must work with symbolic input.

Despite the limitations of the applied artificial intelligence technologies, they are able to provide significant improvements in quality, consistency and productivity making them ideal for product formulation. The technologies discussed in subsequent chapters will deal with:

- Expert (knowledge-based information) systems for formulation.
- Machine learning for rule generation and in case-based reasoning.
- Neural networks for modelling formulations.
- Genetic algorithms for optimising formulations.
- Knowledge discovery in databases.

7

References

BOLD, K., 1989, Expertensysteme unterstutzen bei der Produktformulierung, *Chem. Ztg.*, **113**, 343–346.

CASSON, M., 1983, *The Growth of International Business*, London: Allen and Unwin.

CARTWRIGHT, H.M., 1993, *Application of Artificial Intelligence in Chemistry*, Oxford: Oxford Science Publications.

The New Encyclopaedia Britannica, 1995, *Vol 1. Micropaedia Ready Reference*, Chicago: Encyclopaedia Britannica.

RICH, E., 1983, *Artificial Intelligence*, New York: McGraw-Hill.

TURBAN, E., 1995, *Decision Support Systems and Expert Systems*, 4th edition, Englewood Cliffs, NJ: Prentice-Hall.

2

Expert Systems Fundamentals

2.1 Definition and Structure

There is a wide divergence of opinion as to what defines an expert system. Most definitions can be divided into those that state what an expert system does and those that specify how it works; examples are:

'An expert system is an intelligent computer program that uses knowledge and inference procedures to solve problems that are difficult enough to require significant human expertise for their solutions' (Feigenbaum, 1982).

'An expert system is a knowledge-based system that emulates expert thought to solve significant problems in a particular domain of expertise' (Sell, 1985).

'An expert system is a computer program that assists the user by providing information about a particular domain. It does this by manipulating information about the field that has been provided by a number of experts in the field. Another important feature of an expert system is that it has the facility to explain/justify the methods it used to provide the information' (Doukidis and Whitley, 1988).

'An expert system is a computer program that represents and reasons with knowledge of some specialist subject with a view to solving problems or giving advice' (Jackson, 1990).

'An expert system is a computer program that draws upon the knowledge of human experts captured in a knowledge-base to solve problems that normally require human expertise' (Partridge and Hussain, 1994).

'An expert system is a computer system that applies reasoning methodologies or knowledge in a specific domain in order to render advice or recommendations, much like a human expert' (Turban, 1995).

Because of their emphasis on knowledge, expert systems are also known as knowledge-based or knowledge-based information systems and many authors use the terms interchangeably. In this book the term expert system will be used since, in all the applications discussed later, the input knowledge was acquired from human experts. In systems where knowledge is generally acquired through non-human intervention e.g. via information systems, the term knowledge-based system is more appropriate.

Following on from these definitions is a series of features which Jackson (1990) states are 'sufficiently important that an expert system should really exhibit all of them to some degree':

- It simulates human reasoning about a problem domain, rather than simulating the domain itself.
- It performs reasoning over representations of human knowledge, in addition to doing numerical calculations or data retrieval.
- It solves problems by heuristic or approximate methods which, unlike algorithmic solutions, are not guaranteed to succeed.
- It deals with subject matter of realistic complexity that normally requires a considerable amount of human expertise.
- It must exhibit high performance in terms of speed and reliability in order to be a useful tool.
- It must be capable of explaining and justifying solutions or recommendations to convince the user that its reasoning is in fact correct.

Problem domains addressed by expert systems are many and include (Turban, 1995):

- Prediction i.e. the inference of likely consequences of given situations e.g. weather forecasting.
- Diagnosis i.e. the inference of a system malfunction from observations e.g. medical diagnosis.
- Design i.e. the configuration of objects that satisfy defined constraints e.g. product formulation.
- Interpretation i.e. the inference of situation descriptions from observations e.g. image analysis.
- Planning i.e. the development of actions to achieve goals e.g. product management.
- Repair/correction i.e. the definition of appropriate remedies for a diagnosed problem e.g. solution to problems.
- Monitoring i.e. the comparison of observations to defined targets e.g. air-traffic management.
- Control i.e. the management of the overall behaviour of a system including monitoring and interpreting the current situation, predicting the future, diagnosing the causes of problems and correcting faults e.g. control of any manufacturing process.

Expert systems, in their simplest form, have three components: an interface, an inference engine and a knowledge base. The relationship between these components and the three human elements involved in the development and use of expert systems is shown diagrammatically in Figure 2.1.

For an expert system to be of any use it must be able to communicate with both the user and the developer (knowledge engineer). This is either done directly via a screen and keyboard or indirectly via external links to equipment/machines/

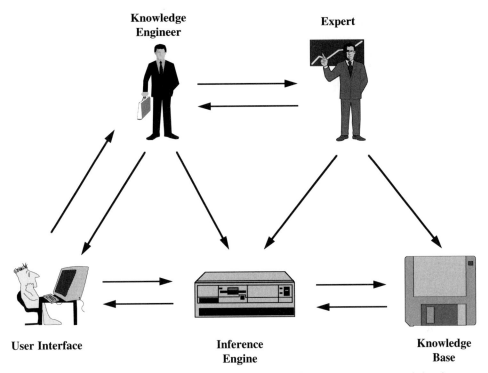

Figure 2.1 The relationship between the components of an expert system and the three human elements involved in its development

monitoring devices. The type of interface will depend on the nature and degree of interaction; the user will generally require an interface that will be easy and friendly to use allowing two way communication as in a question and answer routine, and the knowledge engineer will generally require an interface that is efficient and operational.

In the inference engine, knowledge from the knowledge base is extracted and manipulated and new information generated i.e. the inference engine simulates the process for solving the problem in hand. There are two main approaches for controlling inferencing in rule-based expert systems: forward chaining and backward chaining. The former, often described as data-driven reasoning, is used for problem solving when data or basic ideas obtained from consultation with the user are the starting point. The system then attempts to arrive at conclusions or goals. A problem with forward chaining is that every goal possible is highlighted whether useful or not. In contrast, backward chaining, often described as goal-directed reasoning, starts with a hypothesis or specific goal and then attempts to find data from consultation with the user to prove or disprove the conclusion. Whereas forward chaining is often used in expert systems for design (e.g. product formulation) backward chaining is specifically applicable to diagnostic, control or monitoring systems. However, in most developed systems both inferencing methods are used either singly or combined.

Most inferencing engines also have the ability to reason in the presence of uncertainty both in the input data and also in the knowledge base. The major methods used are Bayesian probabilities and fuzzy logic.

Associated with inferencing is the search mechanism. In many cases it is possible to describe the knowledge base using some kind of tree-like structure. Inferencing then translates into a problem of searching a tree to arrive at an effective solution. A special language has been developed to describe a search tree. The initial state node is called the root node from which other nodes are joined by branches. Nodes with no successions are called the leaf nodes and designate the end of the search. The nodes are divided up into various levels describing the depth of the tree. The root node is usually designated level 0 and successive deeper levels are designated by sequentially higher numbers (Figure 2.2).

There are two strategies commonly used to search such a tree:

- Depth-first search: in which a search is initiated downward along a given path until a solution or dead end is reached. In the latter case the process backtracks to the first alternative branch and tries it. The procedure is repeated until a solution is found (Figure 2.2A).

- Breadth-first search: in which a search is initiated at a specific level on each branch in turn before moving on to a different level (Figure 2.2B).

A depth-first search guarantees a solution but may take a long time. It is particularly useful where branches are short. Breadth-first search routines are useful where the number of branches is relatively small and where the numbers of levels in each branch vary.

Finally, the last and most important component of an expert system is its knowledge base where all the knowledge concerning the domain is stored. The discipline whereby this knowledge is acquired from the experts, structured and represented within the knowledge base is known as knowledge engineering.

2.2 Knowledge Engineering

Knowledge in any domain usually takes the form of facts, rules and heuristics; the facts being the objects and concepts about which the expert reasons, the rules and heuristics (often referred to as rules of thumb) being derived from this reasoning. The difference between rules and heuristics is based on the validity and rigour of the arguments used to justify them – rules are always true, valid and can be justified by rigorous argument; heuristics are the expert's best judgement, may not be valid in all cases and can only be justified by examples.

Associated with these are the terms data and information. Whereas data refers to facts and figures, information is data transformed by processing and organised so that it is meaningful to the person receiving it. Knowledge can therefore be regarded as information combined with heuristics and rules. Even more abstract is wisdom which can be regarded as knowledge tempered by judgement and supplemented by experience and learning (Partridge and Hussain, 1994). These concepts can be classified by their degree of abstraction and by their quantity (Figure 2.3).

There are two levels of knowledge: shallow or surface knowledge and deep knowledge; and three main categories: declarative, procedural and metaknowledge:

- Shallow knowledge, as its name suggests, is a representation of only surface-level information and can only deal with very specific situations.

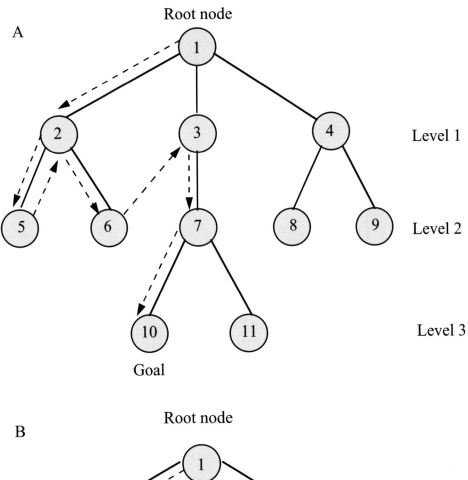

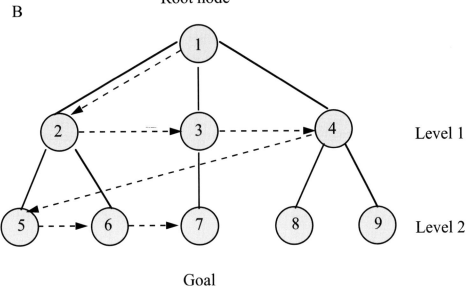

Figure 2.2 Search trees: (A) depth-first search; (B) breadth-first search

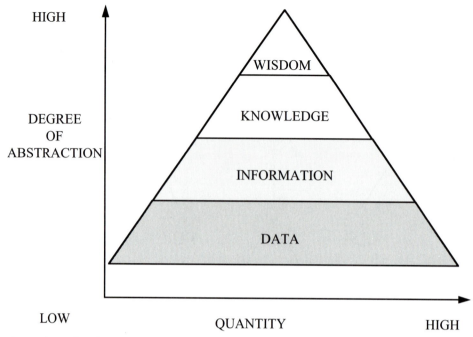

HIGH

DEGREE
OF
ABSTRACTION

LOW   QUANTITY   HIGH

Figure 2.3   The classification of data, information, knowledge and wisdom

- Deep knowledge is a representation of all the information pertaining to a domain. It can include such human characteristics as emotion and intuition and hence is difficult to structure in a computer.
- Declarative knowledge is a descriptive representation of the facts pertaining to a domain and is considered shallow in nature.
- Procedural knowledge is a detailed set of instructions on how to carry out a procedure.
- Metaknowledge is knowledge about knowledge, i.e. knowledge about how a system operates or reasons. It is especially useful in generating explanations.

All of this knowledge about a specific domain is in the form of expertise (often gathered over many years of work) resident with the domain expert or, in the case of large complex domains, a number of experts. It is the objective of the knowledge engineer to acquire or elicit this knowledge from the experts and other sources and structure it in the computer such that it can be used by non-experts.

2.2.1 *Knowledge Acquisition*

The first step in knowledge acquisition is to collect all the potential sources of knowledge (Figure 2.4). These include written documents i.e. books written specifically in the domain, research and technical reports, reference manuals, case studies and even standard operating procedures and organisational policy statements. Availability of written documents varies from case to case; in some domains there may be many available, and in others none at all. Written documents contain

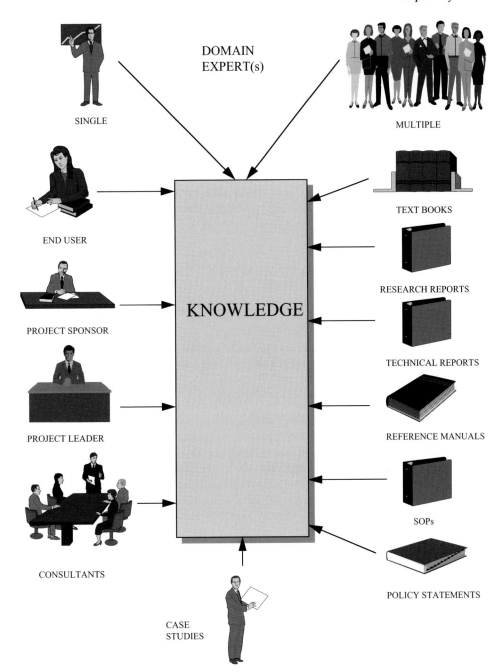

Figure 2.4 Sources of knowledge

factual knowledge; they are often detailed, precise and well structured but are not always relevant for the knowledge acquisition task. However, if significant written documents exist, their exploitation is time and cost effective especially in allowing the knowledge engineer to obtain a broad view of the domain.

Knowledge can also be obtained from discussion with organisational personnel e.g. the project sponsor, the project leader and various consultants. However, the

15

most important source of knowledge is the domain expert or experts. In general two kinds of knowledge may be elicited from these people.

- Explicit knowledge, i.e. knowledge that the domain expert is conscious of having and is able to articulate.
- Tacit knowledge, i.e. knowledge that the domain expert is not conscious of having but does exist as proved by the expert's known capability of solving problems in the application domain.

Explicit knowledge is very easy to elicit from the experts since it is mainly factual in nature. Tacit knowledge is difficult to identify and elicit but is essential for the successful development of expert systems. In eliciting both types of knowledge the knowledge engineer must be aware that all verbal data acquired is often imperfect i.e. knowledge can be:

- incomplete since experts often forget;
- superficial since experts often cannot articulate in detail;
- imprecise since experts may not know the exact detail;
- inconsistent since the experts often fall into contradictions;
- incorrect since experts may be wrong;
- often unstructured since experts often cannot articulate their knowledge in an organised fashion, often jumping from one topic to another.

The decision to employ one or more experts in the knowledge acquisition process is a difficult one since there can be both advantages and disadvantages with this approach. Multiple experts certainly have the advantage of providing a greater distribution of labour, varied opinions/expertise, reducing individual bias but offering a completeness to the knowledge base. However, this can lead to increased costs and disruption to the function. There are often logistical problems in getting everybody together at the same time. In addition varied opinions/expertise and personal incompatibilities can often lead to conflicting viewpoints, difficult to reconcile. For small domains it is often sufficient to use one expert to develop the system but to use others in the evaluation stage. However, for large complex domains multiple experts must be considered.

It can be seen that there are specific characteristics necessary for the domain expert or experts. If the knowledge acquisition process is to be successful the experts must:

- have deep knowledge of the domain;
- be willing to participate in the development of the expert system;
- be convinced of the importance of the project;
- have strong interpersonal skills;
- be allowed time to participate in the project and be supported in this by management at all levels. This is essential since the development of an expert system is time consuming.

Coupled with these are the required skills of the knowledge engineer:

- a deep knowledge of the technology involved in the development of expert systems;

- good communication skills;

- fast learning and logical thinking;

- sensitivity and diplomacy;

- patience and tolerance;

- organised and persistent;

- good interviewing skills.

The last trait is essential since dialogue between the knowledge engineer and expert(s) generally takes the form of face-to-face interviews. However, before this takes place it is helpful if the knowledge engineer has read some of the literature pertaining to the domain and has a basic understanding of it. Some believe that the knowledge engineer should have reached a level of knowledge comparable to that ascribed to the potential users of the finished system. This is not generally a pre-requisite; it may be disadvantageous since it may introduce bias. Certainly special attention needs to be paid by the knowledge engineer to the domain jargon and any acronyms commonly used.

Interviews can be time consuming and tedious, producing large amounts of information. For instance it has been calculated that an expert talking continuously can produce about 10 000 words or 20 pages of transcript per hour. In order to collect such large amounts of information, electronic aids (e.g. tape recorders) can be used but, more often than not, direct transcription as notes generally proves to be the best compromise.

In the interviewing process the expert(s) may be asked to describe a process or problem to the knowledge engineer who will interrupt and ask questions. Some-times the expert may be asked to articulate the solution. Other times the expert may be asked to act as a teacher, tutoring the knowledge engineer in the skills necessary to perform the task.

Interviews can place a great burden on the expert(s) leading to boredom and frustration. Hence it is important for the knowledge engineer to vary the approaches used, structure the interview such that there is a clear objective and generally restrict it to no more than two hours. At all times there must be an empathy between the knowledge engineer and the expert(s) and, in many cases, it is helpful to have two knowledge engineers present at the interview.

A technique often used in the acquisition process is the rapid prototyping approach. In this the knowledge engineer builds a small prototype system as early as possible. This is then inspected by the expert(s) who can then suggest modi-fications and additions. The system then grows incrementally. This approach has certain advantages in that it is possible to demonstrate a system to all parties at an early stage and thus keep their involvement and enthusiasm. However, as the system begins to get larger, it can lose structure and become obscure i.e. there is a loss of the overview of the system. Rapid prototyping is best used when the domain can be broken down into distinct modules.

In addition to these so-called manual methods of knowledge acquisition are the automated methods whereby computers are used. Two methods that have been used in the development of expert systems in the domain of product formulation are rule induction and case-based reasoning. These will be dealt with separately in Chapter 4.

2.2.2 **Knowledge Representation**

A variety of ways of representing knowledge in a knowledge base have been developed over the years. All share two common characteristics: first, they can be programmed and stored in memory; and second, they are described in such a way that they can be manipulated by the inference engine that uses search and inferencing procedures (Section 2.1). The commonly used methods discussed here are production rules, frames, semantic networks, decision tables/trees and objects.

Production rules

These express the relationship between several pieces of information. They are conditional statements that specify actions to be taken or advice to be followed under certain sets of conditions. In its simplest form the production rule is a list of IF clauses followed by a list of THEN clauses:

IF (condition)
THEN (action)

An example of a simple production rule in the formulation of a tablet would be as follows:

IF (drug is insoluble)
THEN (use a soluble filler)

In many expert systems production rules take the more complicated form of:

IF (condition 1)
AND (condition 2)
OR (condition 3)
THEN (action)
UNLESS (exception)
BECAUSE (reason)

For example:

IF (drug is insoluble)
AND (drug is high dose)
OR (drug is hydrophobic)
THEN (use a soluble filler)
UNLESS (drug and filler are incompatible)
BECAUSE (instability will occur)

Both the IF and THEN side of a rule may include several AND/OR operations. Production rules are able to deal with uncertainty using simple probabilities. In this case they can take the form of:

IF (condition) (with probability)
AND (condition) (with probability)
OR (condition) (with probability)
THEN (action) (with certainty)

where probability and certainty are computed factors between 0 and 1 (i.e. 0.4 is equivalent to 40 per cent probability). The confidence with which the action is taken depends on the probability with which each condition holds and the certainty with which the action follows if every condition holds.

For example:

IF (drug is insoluble) (0.9)

AND (drug is high dosage) (0.5)

THEN (use a soluble filler) (CF)

In this example for the action to be true, both the IF statements must be true but there is some uncertainty for this. In such a case the certainty factor (CF) will be 0.5 since this is the minimum probability on the IF side.

However, in the case of an OR operator, a different argument applies.

For example:

IF (drug is insoluble) (0.9)

OR (drug is hydrophobic) (0.5)

THEN (use a soluble filler) (CF)

In this case it is sufficient that only one of the IF statements is true for the action to be true, i.e. the certainty factor (CF) for this rule will be 0.9 since this is the maximum probability on the IF side.

Each production rule implements an autonomous piece of knowledge and can be developed and modified independently of other rules. However, when combined, a set of rules will often yield better results than the sum of the results of the individual rules and independency is lost. This means that extreme care must be taken when adding new rules to a current knowledge base to avoid conflict. Rules called demons are often included in the inference engine. These are actions which are triggered when a certain set of conditions arises. They act as interrupts.

Production rules have several advantages:

- Rules are easy to understand since they are a natural form of knowledge.
- Inference and explanations are derived.
- Rules are able to deal with uncertainty.
- Modification and maintenance are relatively easy.

However, they also have limitations:

- Complex knowledge can require large numbers of rules causing the system to become difficult to manage.
- The production rule format is often inadequate or inconvenient to represent many types of knowledge or to model the structure of specific domains.

Frames

These are a template for holding clusters of related knowledge about a particular object. They are able to represent the attributes of an object in a more descriptive way than is possible using production rules. The frame typically consists of a number of slots which, like attributes, may or may not contain a value. Slots may also

Table 2.1 A frame describing a tablet

Object	Slots	Contents
Tablet	IS-A	Formulation
	Weight	Default 200 mg, actual 203 mg
	Diameter	8 mm actual
	Thickness	If added, check value
	Disintegration time	1–5 minutes range

contain pointers to other frames, sets of rules or procedures by which values may be obtained. The ability to vary slot values contributes greatly to the power of frames. Consider a frame describing a tablet (Table 2.1).

The frame contains a number of different values. The weight slot has both a default and actual value, the diameter has an actual value defined by the die used, the thickness slot has a procedure attached to it. In this case the procedure is called whenever a value is added and checks that it is within reasonable limits. The disintegration time slot has a range of values.

Frames may also be arranged in a hierarchy permitting inheritance of characteristics i.e. each frame inherits the characteristics of all related frames of higher levels in the hierarchy.

Frames have several advantages:

- The ability to document clearly information about a specific object in a domain that consists of several objects.

- The ability to constrain the values of an attribute.

- Ease of maintenance and expansion.

- Access to a mechanism that supports inheritance.

Semantic networks

This is a way of representing complex relationships between objects. It is a network in which descriptors are applied not only to an object or concept (the nodes of the network) but also to their relationship (the lines joining the nodes). A simple network for a tablet formulation is shown in Figure 2.5. In this network the IS-A link is used to define inheritance, and the HAS-A link to connect attributes.

If the links are used to express causation then the network is referred to as a causal network. In this case links can have numeric tags (usually integers) to express the degree of causation i.e. a large positive integer would infer a large positive influence while a small negative integer would infer a small negative influence.

This method of representing knowledge has several advantages:

- It is visual and easy to understand.

- It is flexible allowing easy addition of new nodes and links.

- The network functions in a manner similar to that of human information storage.

- The network has the ability to represent inheritance.

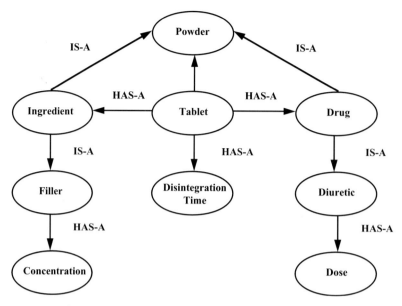

Figure 2.5 A simple semantic network for a tablet

Although semantic networks are represented as pictures they appear in the computer program as statements. Searching large semantic networks can be difficult, hence they are often used for analytical purposes. Causal networks are very useful in a well bounded domain such as product formulation where the connectivity of the network is high and the quantification of causation difficult.

Decision tables/trees

In a decision table knowledge is organised in a spreadsheet format using columns and rows, the columns representing the attributes and the rows representing the conclusion. Once constructed the knowledge in the table can be used as input to other knowledge representation methods. It may also be used for rule induction (Chapter 4).

Decision trees are related to decision tables and can be constructed from them using rule induction algorithms (Chapter 4). A decision tree is composed of nodes representing the goals and links representing decisions i.e. at each node there is an explicit question to answer and the actual answer given determines which of the alternative subsequent nodes is selected at the next decision point.

Decision tables and trees are easy to understand and program. The techniques do not work well for complex systems because they become unwieldy and difficult to interpret.

Objects

An alternative approach to representing knowledge is to use objects, attributes and values. Objects may be physical or conceptual, attributes are the characteristics of the objects and values are the specific measures of the attributes. The difference between objects and frames is that within object-oriented programming

21

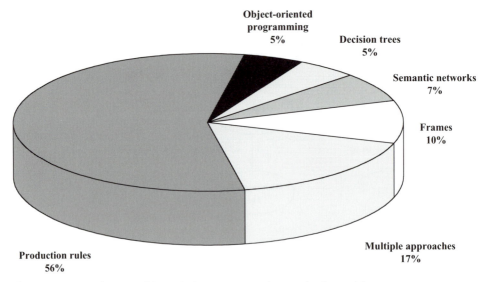

Figure 2.6 Distribution of knowledge representation methods used in expert systems (O'Neill and Morris, 1989)

environments, objects can be regarded as if they were able to act as independent entities. Control of the system is achieved by sending instructions known as messages to the objects and by objects sending and receiving messages between themselves.

The decision as to which method of knowledge representation is used depends very much on the complexity of the domain and the development tool used (Section 2.3). In a survey in 1987/88 of 50 expert systems in the UK, O'Neill and Morris (1989) found a distribution as shown in Figure 2.6. Over one half of the systems were developed using production rules although nearly a sixth used multiple approaches. No data exist for product formulation expert systems.

2.3 Development Tools

Expert systems can be developed using either conventional computing languages, special purpose languages, environments or shells/tools. These may be viewed as a two-dimensional classification with axes of speed of implementation and applicability (Figure 2.7). It should be noted that the boundaries between the groups are often blurred and are only for convenience.

2.3.1 *Conventional Languages*

Conventional languages such as FORTRAN, PASCAL or C have the advantages of wide applicability, being well supported and documented, with full flexibility to create data and knowledge structures. It is possible to customise and make as efficient as possible the control and inference strategies but considerable amounts of time and effort are required to create these facilities. Nevertheless conventional languages are still used, often by academics, in the development of expert systems.

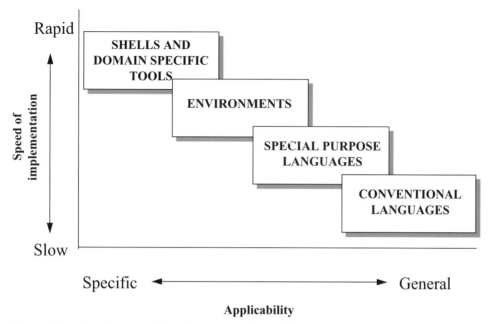

Figure 2.7 Classification of development tools used for expert systems

2.3.2 *Special Purpose Languages*

Special purpose languages include the so called AI or symbolic languages e.g. LISP (LISt Processing) and PROLOG (PROgramming in LOGic) and object-oriented languages e.g. Smalltalk.

LISP is one of the oldest AI languages developed in the USA in 1958. It has been the primary language for AI research in the USA since that time. LISP allows programmers to represent objects like rules, frames and nets as lists or sequences of numbers, character strings or other lists. Lists can be split or joined at random. LISP is a highly interactive, flexible and recursive language ideally suited for many problem solving techniques. With recursion LISP can break large problems into smaller problems where the program calls itself with simplified arguments. These properties allow for elegant solutions to complex problems that are difficult to solve in conventional programming languages. However they do not always make for easily read syntax.

LISP code is usually executed directly by a LISP interpreter. There are numerous variations of LISP, the most commonly used are COMMON LISP, GOLDEN COMMON LISP, INTERLISP and MACLISP.

PROLOG is a language based on first order predicate logic. It was developed in France in 1970 and is the most popular AI language in Europe and Japan. PROLOG is a declarative language in that the user feeds the system facts in predicate form and queries. The system then tries to solve the queries by using the declared knowledge. The declarative nature of the language means that the user specifies constraints to the problem rather than specifying how the problem is to be solved. PROLOG also has the advantage of having a powerful inference engine which uses depth-first searching by backward chaining. Variations of PROLOG include MPROLOG, QUINTUS PROLOG and TURBOPROLOG.

Table 2.2 Some representative examples of environments and their suppliers

Tool	Supplier
ART	Brightware Corp.
KEE	Intellicorp Inc.
Knowledge Craft	Carnegi Group Inc.
AION DS	Platinum Technology Inc.
KBMS	Trinzic Corp.
Nexpert Object	Neuron Data
Goldworks III	Gold Hill Inc.

Object-oriented languages can either be considered as a unique category of programming languages or as a subset of special purpose languages. In essence, object-oriented programming is a decision principle that views descriptive and procedural attributes of an object as being associated with each individual object and hence each object can receive its own messages and perform independent actions. The original object-oriented language was Smalltalk (later versions are now classed as environments); many more are now available e.g. C++, LOOPS, CLOS and Object PASCAL.

2.3.3 *Environments*

Environments can be defined as development systems that support several different ways of representing knowledge and handling inference (Turban, 1995). They may use rules, frames, semantic networks, objects and object-oriented programming, inheritance and different types of chaining. They are more specialised than languages and hence systems can be built more rapidly. Environments are development tools in which interfaces and inference engines can be adapted to suit the needs of the domain.

Environments not only include large commercial systems such as ART, KEE, Knowledge Craft and AION Development System (Table 2.2) (originally defined as large hybrid tools by Harmon *et al.*, 1988) but also the languages Smalltalk and OPS. Smalltalk, originally developed as an object-oriented programming language, has now been expanded to include facilities for data abstraction, object classification and message sending with many built-in graphic interfaces. It is now a complete development system. OPS is a language specially designed for production rule systems. It combines a rule-based language with a conventional procedural programming technique. It should be noted that Knowledge Craft and ART are based on OPS (Harmon *et al.*, 1988).

2.3.4 *Shells/Tools*

Expert system shells are computer programs often written using special programming languages and environments which are capable of being expert systems when loaded with the relevant knowledge. They compromise on applicability/flexibility but this is offset by allowing more rapid development. They offer the basic facilities

Table 2.3 Some representative examples of expert system shells and tools and their suppliers

Tool	Supplier
Crystal	Intelligent Environments Ltd
Exsys	Exsys Inc.
Insight 2+	Level Five Research
Knowledge Pro	Knowledge Garden Inc.
GURU	Micro Data Base Systems
Xi Plus	Brightware Corp.
Kappa-PC	Intellicorp Inc.

of a knowledge base with one or more methods of knowledge representation and an inference engine with one or more inferencing techniques. Shells differ in their secondary characteristics such as user interfaces, operating speeds, the power and flexibility of the language in which the knowledge is represented and the associated algorithmic and arithmetic computational characteristics.

Using this approach expert systems can be built much faster with little programming skill. Shells are very useful for developing expert systems for specific applications. However they do have limitations because of their inflexibility. Examples of some commercial shells are given in Table 2.3. Not included in the list are the so-called domain specific tools. These are designed to be used only in the development of an expert system in a specific domain. Domain specific tools not only contain the facilities of standard shells but also provide specialised development support and user interfaces. Such features permit faster development of applications. A domain specific tool of relevance to product formulation is PFES – Product Formulation Expert System from Logica UK Ltd (Chapter 3).

References

DOUKIDIS, G.I. and WHITLEY, E.A., 1988, *Developing Expert Systems*, Kent: Chartwell-Bratt.

FIEGENBAUM, E.A., 1982, *Knowledge Engineering for the 1980s*, Department of Computer Science, Stanford University.

HARMON, P., MAUS, R. and MORRISSEY, W., 1988, *Expert Systems Tools and Applications*, New York: John Wiley and Sons.

JACKSON, P., 1990, *Introduction to Expert Systems*, 2nd edition, New York: Addison-Wesley.

O'NEILL, M. and MORRIS, A., 1989, Expert systems in the United Kingdom: an evaluation of development methodologies, *Expert Systems*, **6** (2), 90–91.

PARTRIDGE, D. and HUSSAIN, K.M., 1994, *Knowledge-Based Information Systems*, London: McGraw-Hill.

SELL, P.S., 1985, *Expert Systems – A Practical Introduction*, Basingstoke: Camelot Press.

TURBAN, E., 1995, *Decision Support Systems and Expert Systems*, Englewood Cliffs, NJ: Prentice-Hall.

3

Product Formulation Expert System (PFES)

P. BENTLEY
Logica UK Ltd

3.1 Introduction

PFES, Logica's Product Formulation Expert System, is a reusable software kernel and associated methodology to support the generic formulation process. PFES arose from research work in which Logica was involved during the mid-1980s. Since then Logica has developed today's Windows-based product and used it as the basis for a variety of formulation-support tools across a range of industry sectors, most notably pharmaceuticals. PFES is now used operationally in a number of formulation fields such as foods, soft drinks, pet foods, household cleaners, paints, pesticides, etc.

The concept of expert systems is described in Chapter 2. This chapter describes the facilities offered by PFES. To illustrate how PFES can be applied to a formulation domain, a tablet formulation application similar to that developed by Logica for Zeneca Pharmaceuticals has been used for the purposes of illustration. An example of the tablet formulation application produced by this system is shown in Appendix 1.

3.2 History

Today's PFES product arose from research work, as illustrated in Figure 3.1. During the 1980s artificial intelligence (AI), and expert systems in particular, were the subject of much research. At this time specialised software, and sometimes specialised hardware also, were used by researchers in this field. The PFES research project was conducted by a consortium of Shell Research Ltd, Schering Agrochemicals Ltd and Logica UK Ltd under the UK Alvey Programme sponsored by the Department of Trade and Industry (DTI) between 1985 and 1987. This research work investigated the formulation process. Two separate formulation systems in the fields of agrochemicals and lubricating oils were constructed. From these two applications the generic design of PFES was abstracted and a prototype developed. A third application was developed for vinyl coatings (Chapter 8) to validate the

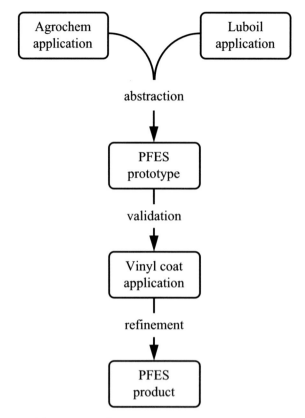

Figure 3.1   History of the PFES product

prototype. The two initial applications, together with PFES itself, were developed using the Knowledge Craft environment from the Carnegi Group Inc. and the language COMMOM LISP on special-purpose computers produced by Symbolics Inc.

It is interesting to note that the project involved seven full time staff at a cost of £860 000. The project was written up as a report to the Alvey Directorate in five volumes (Alvey, 1987).

Following the research project, the PFES prototype was refined by Logica to produce the first version of the PFES product running on a personal computer under DOS. The product remained written in COMMON LISP, but Knowledge Craft was eliminated since it was not available on the PC platform. Several successful applications were developed using this product in the late 1980s and early 1990s. More recently, versions of PFES have been produced for the Apple Macintosh and Microsoft Windows.

3.3   Overview

PFES is designed specifically for building formulation systems. Its formulation capability is generic i.e. it is not specific to any particular domain. Individual formulation applications are developed using PFES by defining characteristics of the domain and the corresponding approach to formulation. The end result is a decision support tool for formulators that provides assistance in all aspects of the formulation development process.

PFES provides the expert system developer with the knowledge representation structures that are common to most product formulation tasks so that a new application can be developed rapidly and efficiently. Development with PFES is therefore likely to be easier than with general purpose expert system shells where the relevant structures for formulation may need to be constructed on top of the tool and irrelevant structures and techniques may introduce unnecessary overheads.

PFES provides a variety of facilities to assist in the development, validation, maintenance and usage of formulation-support systems:

- Facilities are provided to represent the entities, objects and relationships of the formulation application (known as the domain knowledge) in a way which reflects their groupings and associations in the real world. This is essential as a foundation for the problem solving approach (the reasoning process) of the formulation specialist. Existing information sources, such as databases, may need to be represented within the model.

- A method of structuring and representing the problem solving approach of the human formulator is provided. This is critical for the successful representation of the formulation process. The decomposition of the problem solving approach into components which can be explicitly reasoned about and manipulated is important when searching for an approach to take to a particular formulation problem.

- A means of interaction between elements of the problem solving approach is provided. It is important to break the formulation process into a number of discrete elements, in order to focus attention and to provide manageable elements of the problem solving approach which can be reasoned about. Formulation is a sufficiently complex task that these components cannot be made wholly independent (though they are often largely so). It is therefore necessary to have a means of communication information between elements. For example, one element of the problem solving process may result in certain preferences which should be taken into account by subsequent problem solving elements. Hence, the identified preferences need to be communicated from one problem solving element to another.

- A means of specifying the formulation problem to be solved and of making that specification accessible to the problem solving knowledge is supplied. The specification of the formulation problem is the input to the formulation process, and so it is important to be able explicitly to represent and to reason about the specification. The specification may need to be modified during the course of the formulation process.

- The formulation itself is explicitly represented as it is refined from beginning to end of the formulation process. The formulation is the output from the formulation process and must be built up and made more specific as the problem solving process proceeds.

- Supporting the exploration of different formulation routes during the formulation development process is provided. A way to consider a number of options concurrently is provided. A choice among the options will be made when each has been investigated to a sufficient extent.

- The suspension of formulation problems, pending the arrival of more information. Many formulation development processes have long elapse times, for instance while tests or trials are underway.

- Monitoring facilities and explanation. PFES keeps the formulator informed of the progress on the formulation problem, and the formulator can find out what factors were taken into account in arriving at a recommendation. This is vital for most of the roles identified above.

3.4 Features

The PFES software embodies many features which together provide an efficient and effective environment.

The interactive environment allows the formulator to suspend the formulation process in order to examine the current state and even to wind the process backwards so that an alternative strategy can be investigated.

The dynamic view of the ongoing formulation process provides visibility of the status of the process and significant information relating to it. The status of the process is revealed by a window showing the tasks which have been completed, the one which is current, and those which are still to be done. These tasks are indented to reflect their position in the hierarchy. An example is shown in Figure 3.2. The current state of the specification and the formulation itself are also shown in their own windows, as shown in Figure 3.3.

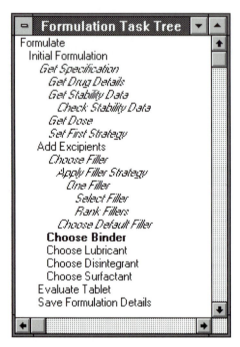

Figure 3.2 The PFES Formulation Task Tree window showing the current status of the formulation process for a tablet formulation. Tasks in italics have been completed, and the one in bold is currently running

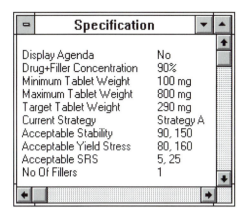
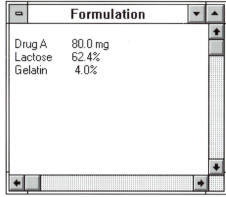

Figure 3.3   The PFES Specification and Formulation windows showing the current status of the corresponding entities of specification and formulation

Sodium Starch Glycolate

Exit	*Disintegrant*
is a	Disintegrant
YP	40.3
YP Fast	79.5
SRS	97.3
Trade Name	Primojel
	Explotab
Efficiency Rating	10
Initial Level	0.04

Figure 3.4   A knowledge browser window showing what is known about the tablet disintegrant sodium starch glycolate

A PFES application includes a database which typically includes information on active agents (e.g. drugs) and ingredients (e.g. excipients) used in the formulation process. This database is described in the next section. A powerful browsing facility allows the formulator to examine the contents of the database simply by selecting entries which are of interest. For instance, if an excipient name is chosen, not only are the properties of that excipient displayed, but all references to the excipient from elsewhere in the database are also retrieved. Figures 3.4 and 3.5 show example knowledge browser windows.

Knowledge editors are an integral part of PFES. These are used to develop and maintain the knowledge encapsulated in an application. The editors are easy to use, being menu driven to avoid the need to understand details such as syntax. Access to the editors can be protected by passwords to prevent unauthorised modifications.

Often data concerning active agents and ingredients are already available in machine-readable form (typically spreadsheets or databases). These data can be directly imported to PFES, ensuring that the data used are consistent and up to date.

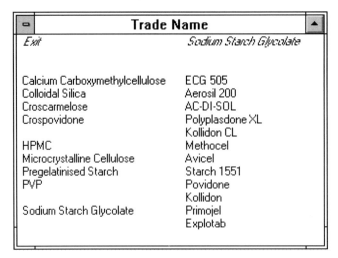

Figure 3.5   A knowledge browser window showing all the excipient trade names in the database for the tablet disintegrant sodium starch glycolate

Other features of PFES include:

- A Help facility which can be extended to cover details of the application. This facility is usually used to provide background information and guidance on how to use a particular application. It has also been utilised to provide support for training formulators.

- The encryption of the application files stored on disk in order to protect the embodied knowledge and data which are often commercially sensitive.

- An automatic rule checker which ensures that all rules are properly formed.

3.5   Knowledge Structure

The architecture of PFES comprises three levels, as illustrated in Figure 3.6: the Physical Level, Task Level and the Control Level.

3.5.1   *Physical Level*

The Physical Level contains all the 'nuts and bolts' of the formulation domain in a number of information sources. The Physical Level is accessed from the Task Level via a query interface.

The physical net contains the domain knowledge in a number of objects. An object consists of a set of attributes, each of which may have zero or more values. The objects are arranged in a classification hierarchy. Sub-objects which descend from another object inherit its attributes and their values.

Figure 3.7 provides an illustration of an object hierarchy for the excipients used in a tablet formulation. 'Filler', 'Binder', etc. are all sub-objects (sub-classes) of 'Excipient'. They therefore inherit all properties (attributes and their values) of 'Excipient', thus ensuring that each has a similar representation. Mannitol is an instance of a 'Filler'. It has three attributes:

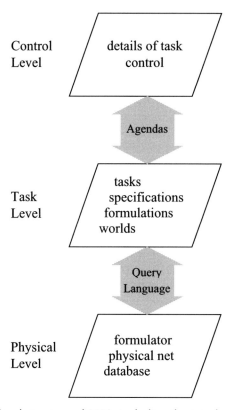

Figure 3.6 The three-level structure of PFES, including the interfaces between the levels. Some of the important components are listed within each level

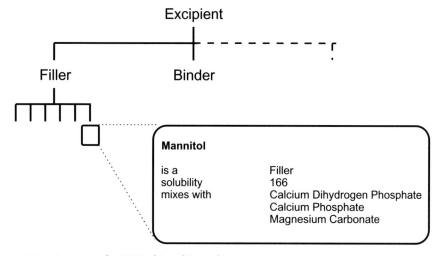

Figure 3.7 An example PFES object hierarchy

- Is a: the immediate classification of the excipient (Filler). This is meant to be read as 'mannitol is a filler'. Due to the hierarchy, mannitol is also (indirectly) classified as an 'Excipient'.

- Solubility: the solubility of mannitol, here represented numerically (166 mg ml^{-1}). Alternatively, the solubility could have been represented symbolically (e.g. freely soluble).

- Mixes with: the set of other fillers (calcium dihydrogen phosphate, calcium phosphate, magnesium carbonate) with which mannitol is known to be used as mixtures.

The 'is a' attribute is common to all objects in the Physical Level. Sometimes it has multiple values reflecting the fact that some excipients serve several roles. For example, maize starch can be classified as a binder, disintegrant and filler. The 'solubility' attribute (though not its value) is inherited from 'Excipient' reflecting the fact that all excipients will have a solubility (though for each the actual value is different). The 'mixes with' attribute is defined at the 'Filler' level since, in this application, the only class of excipient for which compatible instances are sought is for fillers.

3.5.2 Task Level

The Task Level is where the formulation problem solving activity takes place. The formulation process is driven via the generation of a hierarchy of tasks. A task conforms to the common English usage of the word; it represents some well defined activity. There is an indefinite number of levels of tasks in the hierarchy. A fragment of a task hierarchy is shown in Figure 3.8; an example PFES display in

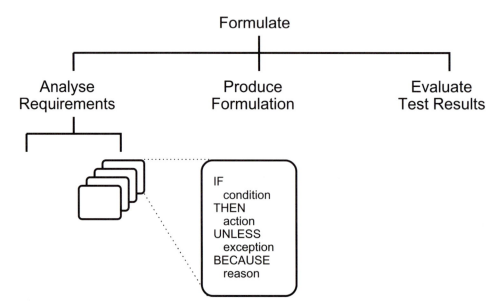

Figure 3.8 A PFES task hierarchy including a rule template

Figure 3.2. Domain knowledge about the formulation application is distributed throughout the hierarchy, with more abstract knowledge represented towards the top of the hierarchy and more specific knowledge towards the bottom.

The task decomposition allows the problem solving process to be largely decoupled between tasks and also facilitates reasoning about sub-tasks. An important principle is that tasks plan about and directly manipulate only their immediate sub-tasks. Recursive application of this principle is the key to integrated behaviour of a formulation system as a whole. The task tree is built on dynamically, depending on the specification in hand, as the problem solving process proceeds. This is different to the object hierarchy where the structure is fixed for a particular domain.

In the Task Level there is a particularly important class of object used for communication between tasks called agendas. One of the reasons for the importance of agendas is that the user exercises control over the formulation process principally through agenda manipulation. Two other objects in the Task Level are the formulation object and the specification object, examples of which are shown in Figure 3.3. These objects are the repositories of all the formulation variables, where a formulation variable is any property associated with the formulation which can be given a value or constrained during the formulation process. The formulation object contains any formulation variable which is a component, and represents the current composition of the formulation. The specification object holds all other formulation variables, for example process temperature or application type, and hence represents the current state of knowledge about the formulation problem. There may be several formulation and specification objects if several formulation options are being explored.

For parallel reasoning and back-tracking by the user it is necessary to maintain more than one world. A world contains a formulation object and specification object together with agendas, in other words a complete description of the state of the formulation process at any one time. Tasks run on a world or set of worlds; it is meaningless for tasks to run without reference to worlds.

Tasks perform their function by the execution of processes. Each task contains several types of process. The pre-condition process assesses whether or not the task can play a sensible role in the current context. The action process performs the primary work of the task, which can include scheduling sub-tasks to be run next. The monitor process executes between each sub-task, typically to assess their result. Finally, the post-condition process assesses the success of the task as a whole immediately prior to completion.

Each process consists of a set of rules. Rules in PFES have the general form:

IF (condition)

THEN (action)

UNLESS (exception)

BECAUSE (reason)

A rule is said to fire if its condition is true and its exception is false. When a rule fires its action is executed. The reason is for information only and is not interpreted by PFES.

The simplest form of basic rule is the IF (true) rule, which will always allow the THEN clause(s) to fire. This is used for specifying, for instance, default choices:

IF (true)

THEN (add lubricant to the formulation)

BECAUSE (always need a lubricant)

Here is an example rule to determine whether a surfactant is required in a tablet formulation by reasoning about the contact angle of the drug:

IF (drug has value <drug> in the formulation)

AND (contact angle has value <angle> in <drug>)

AND (<angle> is greater than 80°)

THEN (add surfactant to the formulation)

BECAUSE (include surfactant when contact angle > 80°)

Repeated clauses in the IF and THEN parts are implicitly combined with a logical AND operation, whereas UNLESS clauses are combined with OR (Chapter 2). Variables are allowed in rules and are contained within angular brackets <>. Variables will be bound if they appear in the condition or exception of the rule and can be referenced again in the action part. If the condition fails or the exception succeeds then further bindings of variables are tried (via back-tracking) until the rule fires or no more bindings are available.

Rules are assigned a priority reflecting the order in which they should be considered. When executing a rule-set, rules are tried in order until no more rules can fire. To find a suitable rule PFES orders the rules first on priority and then on specificity. The first rule having a true condition and false exception is fired, and its action executed. The process of finding the next rule that can fire then starts all over again. To avoid looping, rules are only allowed to fire once with the same set of variable bindings.

For each rule firing, a rule trace is created recording the variable bindings in force. This rule trace is accessible from the user interface.

3.5.3 *Control Level*

The Control Level is concerned with the mechanics of running the Task Level. It contains no domain knowledge and requires no design amendment when a new formulation system is built. Although the Task Level decides which tasks need running and the order in which they should run, the Control Level deals with the mechanics of actually running them and of passing control to them.

3.6 Functionality

The typical functionality of a completed PFES application is as follows:

1   The user enters the product specification which forms the starting point of the formulation. In the tablet formulation example this consists of the drug details (unless already known to the system) and the dose.

2   PFES steps through a series of tasks which select ingredients and determine their quantities based on the product specification. PFES achieves this by following

the rules and other knowledge that have been built into the system during development. An initial formulation is produced.

3   If the system performs reformulation in addition to producing initial formulations, then the user can enter the results of tests that have been performed on the product. PFES will then determine what kinds of problems with the formulation are indicated by the test results. The user can agree with the system's analysis of the problems or modify them as he or she sees fit. PFES uses the problem summary to make recommendations about what ingredients need to be added or what quantities need to be altered, and again the user can override the recommendations if he or she wishes. Once the user is happy with the recommendations PFES will produce a modified formulation which meets the new requirements.

At any point during a session the user can ask for an explanation of the results, browse the system's knowledge, or revert to an earlier stage of the process to modify the specification and obtain another formulation. The user can also save formulations (along with their associated product specifications) and generate printed reports.

3.7   Support for Formulation Development Process

Figure 3.9 illustrates the stages in the formulation development process. The process is cyclic since several iterations are often required before a successful formulation is achieved.

PFES can provide support throughout the formulation development process:

- Analysis of requirements. Before the process of producing a formulation can properly begin it is often necessary to analyse the requirement, possibly seeking further information, and establish the resultant targets and constraints on the formulation. The approach to requirements analysis is similar to that of formulation and therefore is well within the capabilities of PFES.

- Initial formulation and reformulation. Only rarely is a final formulation produced at the first attempt, although this is perhaps the ultimate objective of a sophisticated formulation support system. Therefore, it is usually necessary to refine early attempts successively until a successful result is achieved. In some formulation domains, genuine initial formulations (derived from scratch) are rare; rather the starting point for a new formulation is some similar formulation produced previously. Therefore, PFES applications which support such an

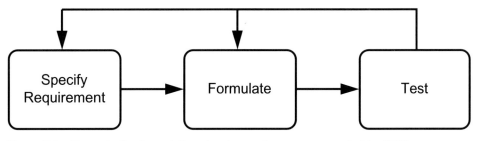

Figure 3.9   Stages in the formulation development process supported by PFES

approach only need provide a reformulation capability. In such instances, this is usually complemented by the capability to search a library of existing formulations for candidates that match the new requirement which can form the starting point. The criteria for such a search typically involve the properties of the formulation rather than the formulation itself.

- Evaluation of test results. In order to assess the adequacy of a formulation, tests on samples have to be performed. Some tests may be avoided if it is possible to predict their results mathematically. In such instances, PFES can be programmed to compute the results, or better still, the desired results can be targeted as part of the formulation process in order that the required properties can be achieved. Nevertheless, some laboratory tests are usually required. PFES can recommend which tests need to be performed, together with the testing methodology where appropriate, based on the requirement specification and the maturity of the formulation. When the tests have been completed the results are provided to PFES. These results are then used to assess the adequacy of the formulation, target any refinements and address deficiencies.

- Providing a database of ingredients, processes, etc. Since information pertinent to the formulation process, such as ingredients (and their properties) is required, PFES can act as a repository for this information. Alternatively, if databases containing such information already exist, the necessary data can be extracted for use by PFES.

- Maintaining a history of formulation development. In order to support the whole formulation process the data arising at each stage are either produced by PFES (e.g. the formulation) or have to be provided to PFES (e.g. test results). PFES can therefore act as a central repository for such information, recording it to establish a complete history of formulation development.

3.8 Complex Formulations

Throughout this chapter reference is made to the ultimate goal of producing a formulation. In fact this is a simplification of reality in two ways, as described below.

Often, due to the uncertainty involved, several formulations are produced at each stage in the development process. The formulations are likely to differ from each other only to a small extent, perhaps the level of a single ingredient. The objective of producing multiple formulations is to explore, in parallel, numerous minor variations where it is not possible to predict the outcome accurately. Each formulation will be evaluated and the best (according to some criteria) selected for subsequent development. PFES supports this manner of working. It allows multiple formulations to be derived concurrently and, following testing, applies the selection criteria to identify which is best. Should this subsequently prove unworkable, an earlier attempt can be reverted to and development recommence again from there.

The focus of a formulation is a list of ingredients and corresponding amounts. However, the output from a formulation support system may consist of more than this. Often other properties relating to the formulation can be computed or estimated, such as strength and shelf life. More significantly, the means of producing the formulation may be equally (or even more) important. In some cases the production process and the formulation itself are interdependent, so one cannot be derived without the other. For instance, with tablet formulation, the type of production process (wet granulation, direct compression, etc.) influences the formulation. PFES applications often derive properties of a formulation and take account of the type of production process to be employed. In some instances detailed production processes are produced alongside the formulation and these may prove to be equally complex.

3.9 Development Life Cycle

Development of a PFES application follows an iterative life cycle whereby the findings from each knowledge acquisition session are rapidly encoded within PFES and then shown to the formulator for refinement. This ensures that the formulator obtains early feedback on how his or her knowledge is reflected in the system's performance in case the result is not what was intended. It also allows the formulator to re-establish the priorities for the project on a regular basis as more is understood about the desired functionality.

Each iteration consists of the following cycle (Figure 3.10):

1   Elicitation – knowledge acquisition session.
2   Implementation – rapid incorporation of new knowledge into prototype.
3   Review – demonstration of prototype to formulator for comment and refinement.

The initial cycles in the development process focus on specific features of the system, while later cycles aim to refine the knowledge and hence the performance of the system.

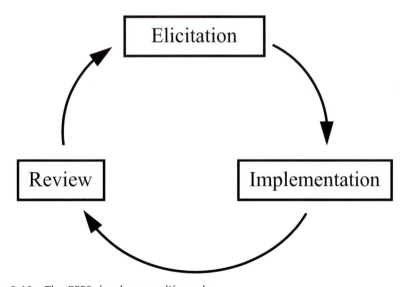

Figure 3.10   The PFES development life cycle

The first stage of development is to identify the product specification that the formulator uses as the starting point for his or her activities and develop the part of the system that asks the user to enter this product specification. The second stage is to enumerate and classify the ingredients that are used in a formulation and to build some very general rules about the amount of each ingredient that is typically used.

The third stage is typically the most time consuming part of the development. In this stage, which usually takes a number of iterations, the detailed rules which map the product specification into an appropriate formulation are added to the system tasks. The number and complexity of the rules depends on the range of parameters in the product specification and on the number of possible ingredients.

Once the system is able to produce a reliable first pass formulation, a possible additional step is to add new knowledge regarding reformulation. This is usually a major step which involves adding a whole new set of objects, tasks and rules.

The final stage is to include additional features to make the system more usable and/or powerful. The precise nature of these features varies between applications but might include generating reports of the formulation session; adding other types of knowledge which impact on the formulation, such as manufacturing knowledge; or creating new input and display capabilities. These features may also be added at any stage during the system development as the need is identified.

The iterative nature of the development means that it is normal to revisit earlier stages in the life cycle at any point in the development, as both developers and formulators gain a better understanding of the reasoning behind the formulation process. Revisiting a stage may involve anything from minor changes to the knowledge to major modifications of the system functionality. Even when the system has reached a stable and useful state, there are some aspects of the knowledge that will need maintaining over time and some enhancements that will be identified as a result of system usage. A good initial design can improve the maintainability and extensibility of the system considerably.

The use of PFES has resulted in extremely efficient development cycles. Turner (1991) has reported that typically demonstration systems can be developed in an organisation's own formulation area with less than 20 man days of consultancy support. Pilot systems can be developed usually with a further 30 to 50 man days of effort. These figures have been confirmed by both Wood (1991) for the development of an application for suncare products and Rowe (1993) for the development of an application for tablets. Some organisations have developed subsequent PFES applications with no further outside help while others prefer to retain specialist consultancy support.

3.10 Conclusion

Logica's Product Formulation Expert System is an advanced software tool designed to improve formulation. Operating on a personal computer it provides a decision support framework which structures the product knowledge and contains information about the formulation process. It has been used extensively in the development of applications for foods, soft drinks, pet foods, household cleaners, paints, pesticides and pharmaceuticals including tablets, capsules and parenterals. Several of these applications are described in detail in Chapters 8 and 9.

References

ALVEY PROJECT REPORT, 1987, IKBS/052, *Product Formulation Expert System*, Vol. 1, The PFES Project; Vol. 2, Description of Applications; Vol. 3, The Formulation Kernel; Vol. 4, The Public Demonstrator; Vol. 5, Recommended Applications and Methodology, London: DTI.

ROWE, R.C., 1993, An expert system for the formulation of pharmaceutical tablets, *Manufacturing Intelligence*, **14**, 13–15.

TURNER, J., 1991, Product Formulation Expert System, *Manufacturing Intelligence*, **8**, 12–14.

WOOD, M., 1991, Expert systems save formulation time, *Lab-Equipment Digest*, December, 17–19.

4

Rule Induction and Case-Based Reasoning

4.1 Introduction

The knowledge acquisition methods presented in Chapter 2 can be time consuming, expensive and often difficult to manage. In some cases, they can, through failure, cause the rejection of expert system development in a company. Technologies that can alleviate this so-called knowledge acquisition bottleneck are Rule induction and Case-based reasoning.

4.2 Rule Induction

Rule induction is a technique that generalises training examples in the form of a knowledge matrix of attributes, properties, values and clauses from which it automatically extracts information in the form of a set of rules or a decision tree. In both cases the knowledge acquired is then used to solve new problems.

Inductive methods use various algorithms to convert the knowledge matrix into either decision trees or rules. Probably the best known of all the tree generating algorithms is ID3 (Quinlan, 1986). ID3 starts with a set of training examples at the root node of the tree. It then selects an attribute to partition the examples. For each value of the attribute a branch is created and a subset of examples that have the attribute value specified by the branch are moved to the newly created node. The algorithm is applied recursively at each of these nodes until either all the examples at a node are of the same class or all the examples have the same values for all the attributes. Every leaf node in the decision tree then represents a classification rule. At each node the algorithm chooses that attribute which provides the maximum degree of discrimination between classes i.e. the tree is constructed in such a way that the information gained by each partitioning is maximal.

Trees generated using ID3 are not necessarily binary in form i.e. the number of branches emanating from each node does not have to be two. ID3 is also very efficient on large data sets generating decision trees that are well balanced i.e. few questions need to be asked before reaching a conclusion. Other variants of the ID3 algorithm are the C4 and C4.5 algorithms (Quinlan, 1993).

Table 4.1   Some representative examples of rule induction tools and their suppliers

Tool	Supplier
1st Class	Trinzic Corp.
VP Expert	World Tech Systems Inc.
Ex-Tran 7	Intelligent Terminals Ltd
SuperExpert	Software Inc.
Level 5	Information Builders
TIMM	General Research
Rule Master	Radian Corp.
Crystal Induction	Intelligent Environments Ltd
KATE Induction	AcknoSoft

The basic ID3 algorithm is present in many induction software tools (Table 4.1). Some (e.g. 1st Class) can also use backward and forward chaining inferencing to generate rule-based expert systems. Others (e.g. KATE Induction) can also handle complex data represented by structural objects with relations and can use background knowledge.

It is interesting to compare the inductive approach with a rule-based expert system created by interviewing experts. This has been done by Perray (1990) using the KATE Induction tool for a credit assessment application with 735 training examples described by 40 numeric and symbolic attributes. The two approaches were evaluated by four experts with 300 new examples not used for induction. The results are shown in Figure 4.1. It can be seen that while both the rule induction and rule-based expert system approaches were not as good as the experts themselves, the induction approach gave significantly less incorrect results than the rule-based expert system. In addition, induction enabled delivery of the application in significantly less time (14 days compared to 60 days).

Despite these results and the obvious advantages of not needing knowledge engineers to develop a system, several difficulties exist with the implementation of rule induction:

- Only classification (including identification) problems can be addressed.

- Experts are still necessary to define the original knowledge matrix and define the attributes.

- The decision tree and rules generated may not be easy to understand because the method by which the induction algorithms classify the attributes and values may not be the same as that used by the expert.

- The larger the set of training examples the better.

- The method is non-incremental. All training examples are used simultaneously in the construction of the decision tree. When new examples become available it is necessary to construct a new tree.

Nevertheless, rule induction is used extensively in the generation of rule-based expert systems if only for the rapid construction of prototypes which can then be translated into more robust systems.

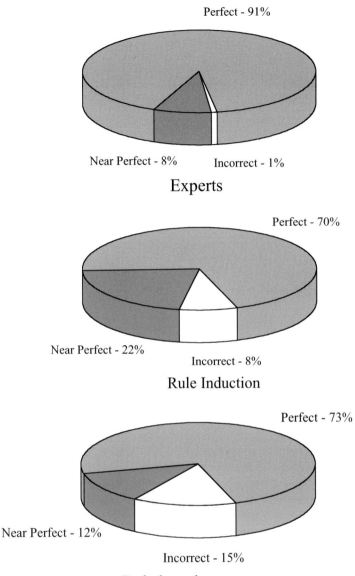

Perfect - 91%

Near Perfect - 8%   Incorrect - 1%

Experts

Perfect - 70%

Near Perfect - 22%

Incorrect - 8%

Rule Induction

Perfect - 73%

Near Perfect - 12%

Incorrect - 15%

Rule based expert system

Figure 4.1 Comparative study between rule induction and a rule-based expert system (results taken from Perray, 1990). Perfect = answer exactly as provided by experts, Near perfect = right answer with a probability above 0.6

In the domain of product formulation, 1st Class has been used both for rule induction for an expert system for the formulation of propellants (Shaw and Fifer, 1988) and in the generation of an expert system for the identification and solution of defects in the film coating applied to pharmaceutical tablets (Chapter 9). In the latter the domain was initially divided into several modules for which individual decision trees were created. These were then linked together and a hypertext system added to create a viable expert system of use in product development (Rowe and Upjohn, 1993).

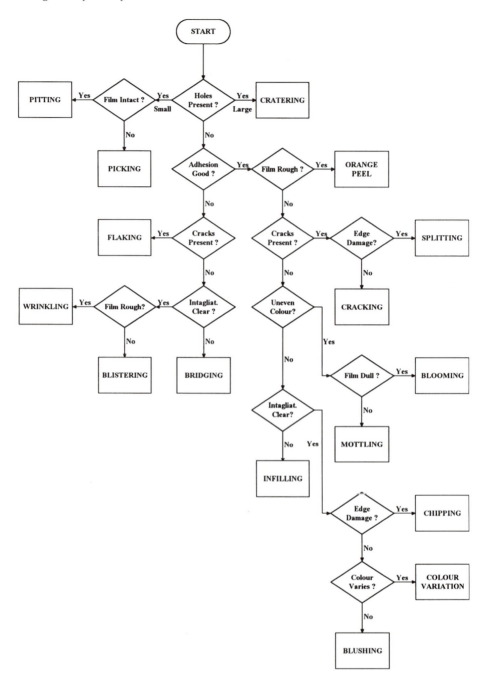

Figure 4.2 A decision tree for the identification of defects on film coated tablets (Rowe and Upjohn, 1993)

Figure 4.2 shows the decision tree generated for this system using ID3 and created to identify a specific defect in a film coated tablet from a possible list of 16 defects. It can be seen that in all but one node the tree is binary in form. This is because it is meant to simulate a question and answer routine between an expert and a novice formulator generally requiring the answer yes or no. Correct identification of the defect at this stage is essential if a correct solution is to be found (Rowe and Upjohn, 1993).

Rule induction of the type described can only be used to describe classes of examples that are already known to exist. In large databases where there may be a large number of examples and less knowledge of the domain it would be advantageous to have a software tool that could discover the classes as well as inducing the rules. This is the approach used in Data Mining or Knowledge Discovery in Databases, where tools have been developed that combine statistics, cluster analysis and rule induction on large databases. This technology will be dealt with later (Chapter 7).

4.3 Case-Based Reasoning

Case-based reasoning (CBR) has recently been described as 'one of those rare technologies whose principles can be explained in a single sentence: to solve a problem, remember a similar problem you have solved in the past and adapt the old solution to solve the new problem' (Goodall, 1995). Case-based reasoning uses directly records of previous solutions (both successful and unsuccessful) to termed cases as its principal knowledge base rather than rules abstracted from them (Figure 4.3). This model of problem solving is one that many experts (including product formulators) use intuitively. Indeed they often talk about their domain by giving examples rather than articulate their knowledge using logical rules.

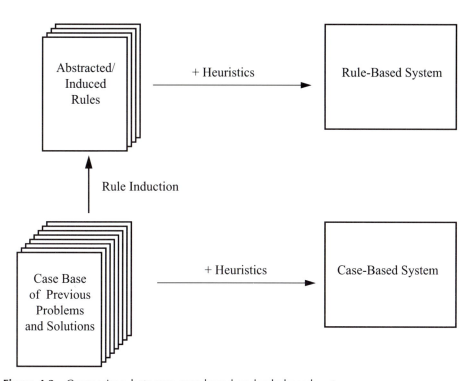

Figure 4.3 Comparison between case-based and rule-based systems

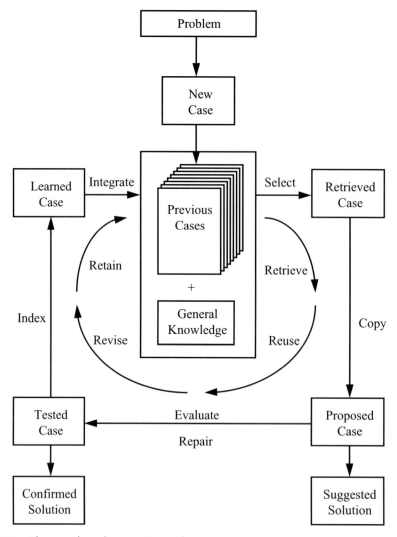

Figure 4.4   The case-based reasoning cycle

The cased-based reasoning cycle can be described by the 4Rs (Aamodt and Plaza, 1994) (see Figure 4.4):

- RETRIEVE the case or cases in memory that give solutions to the problem(s) similar to the current problem.
- REUSE the knowledge about that case to suggest a solution or solutions.
- REVISE and adapt the previous solution(s) to the new problem.
- RETAIN the solution in the memory for future problem solving.

These four main tasks have been sub-divided into other tasks (Aamodt and Plaza, 1994) as shown in Figure 4.5. In order to understand the issues relative to case-based reasoning it is pertinent to discuss these tasks along with case representation.

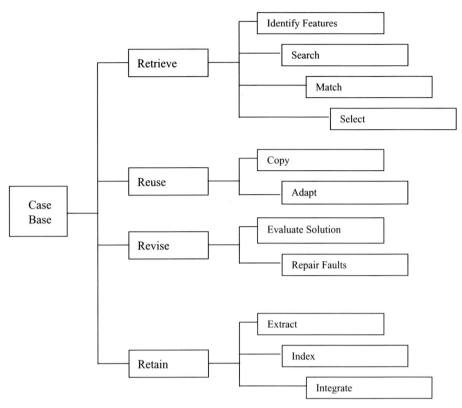

Figure 4.5 Sub-tasks for case-based reasoning

4.3.1 *Case Representation*

Case-based reasoning is dependent on the structure and content of its cases. Cases can be regarded as having three features: a description, an associated solution and a justification of its solution. Justifications are an explicit representation of the process used to solve the problem and can vary in complexity. Cases can be represented using a variety of techniques e.g. frames, semantic networks, and objects with attributes which can be symbolic or numeric. A feature specific to case-based reasoning is the use of indexing, an index being a subset of attributes characterising that case. This feature is necessary to speed up case retrieval.

4.3.2 *Case Retrieval*

The retrieval process involves identifying those features in the new case which best match those in the case base. Identification in a case may simply involve noticing its attributes and indexes and matching these against those in the case base by computing the similarity between the two. Most practical case-based reasoning methods rely on either nearest neighbour based algorithms (clustering algorithms well known in the field of statistics) or induction with decision trees to assess the similarity – the former uses a numerical similarity measure, the latter an exact match against a description.

For a set of similar cases identified a best match is selected. This can be done using similarity measures but more often than not further ranking is necessary and may involve interaction with the user.

4.3.3 *Case Reuse*

In some very simple domains, the solution of the retrieved case may be directly used to solve the new problem. Generally, this does not happen and the old solution will need to be modified or adapted to suit the new problem. There are two ways to reuse past cases: to reuse the solution of the past case – transformational reuse; and to reuse the past method that constructed the solution – derivational reuse.

4.3.4 *Case Revision*

Case revision consists of two tasks, evaluation and fault repair. In the former, the solution may be evaluated by testing or by asking an expert. If the result is a failure then the solution needs to be corrected. Case repair involves deleting the errors of the current solution and retrieving or generating explanations for them. In some developed systems causal knowledge is used to generate explanations. These are then used to modify the solution and the revised case is re-evaluated.

4.3.5 *Case Retainment*

If the solution is satisfactory, information needs to be extracted possibly by adding an explanation or by the construction of a whole new case. If it is the latter, indexes will need to be assigned before integrating the solution into the case base. Failures may also be extracted and retained, either as separate failure cases or within a successful case as an explanation.

The dynamic addition of new knowledge by the addition of new solutions to the case base means that case-based reasoning is intrinsically a learning methodology such that the performance of a system based on this approach will improve with time and the accumulation of experience. This provides distinct advantage as illustrated in one of the first commercially fielded systems initiated in 1987 by Lockheed in Palo Alto, California (Hennessy and Hinkle, 1992).

Known as CLAVIER, its domain is the configuration of autoclave loads for curing composite parts. In the aerospace industry, designing a successful configuration is complicated and time consuming. Successful loads must maximise the number of parts while meeting engineering constraints and minimising time. Each part has its own heating characteristics and parts often interact to alter the heating and cooling characteristics of the autoclave. The internal thermodynamics of the autoclave are complex and, as yet, there is no model to work on. As a result, operators used drawings of earlier successful configurations and adapted them to new requirements. For any new load, CLAVIER uses case-based reasoning to search its case base. If it cannot find an exact match, it takes the stored configuration that most closely matches the current situation and adapts it by finding suitable substitutes for

Table 4.2 Some representative examples of case-based reasoning tools and their suppliers

Tool	Supplier
CBR2	Inference Ltd
ESTEEM	Esteem Software Inc.
CASECRAFT	AcknoSoft
RECALL	ISoft SA
REMIND	Cognitive Systems Inc.
	Intelligent Applications Ltd
S³-CASE	techInno GmbH

the unmatched parts from other successful configurations. Having established what it considers to be the most appropriate configuration, CLAVIER presents it to the operator with justifications. If accepted, the new configuration is added to the case base for future reference. Since September 1990, when the system was installed, the case base has grown from 20 successful configurations to several hundred, resulting in a successful configuration 90 per cent of the time (Keen, 1993).

In addition to being a learning methodology, case-based reasoning has several other advantages:

- Almost limitless applications in domains where there are many exceptions to rules and where problems are not fully understood but where there is a database of past examples. This is often the case in large companies where notebooks are full of examples both successful and unsuccessful.

- The more rapid implementation of expert systems. Past experience with case-based reasoning has shown an 85 per cent reduction in development time with increased accuracy of 30 per cent when compared to other approaches (Keen, 1993).

- The development of a corporate memory.

For a comprehensive text on case-based reasoning the reader is referred to Kolodner's excellent book on the subject (Kolodner, 1993). In addition to analysing a broad range of approaches, the author provides guidelines for building case-based expert systems as well as a comprehensive library of developed case-based reasoning systems.

Several commercial case-based reasoning tools are now available (Table 4.2). As for rule-based system shells these tools can assist in the development of rapid application but at the expense of flexibility of representation, reasoning approach and learning methodology. All these tools have recently been extensively evaluated (Althoff *et al.*, 1995). Despite the availability of these tools, case-based reasoning has not yet specifically been applied to product formulation. However, one successful academic system, appropriately named CHEF, with a domain of Szechwan cooking (Hammond 1986, 1989) can be considered to be a direct analogy to product formulation and will be discussed later (Chapter 8).

In the context of product formulation, a case would be a description of a specific formulation together with its properties, processing method and details of how and why it was developed. The general case-based reasoning approach to creating a new formulation would therefore be:

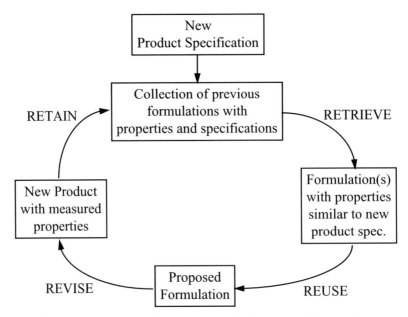

Figure 4.6   The case-based reasoning cycle as applied to product formulation

1   Accepting the specification for the new product.
2   Matching the specification against the properties of any stored formulations.
3   Selecting the stored formulation(s) most relevant to the new specification.
4   Adapting the selected formulation(s) as necessary.
5   Evaluating the new formulation(s).
6   Storing the new formulation(s) and properties in the case base.

This is a typical Retrieve, Reuse, Revise, Retain cycle (Figure 4.6) and it is only a matter of time before it is used to create new products.

As with rule induction case-based reasoning has become one of the underlying technologies in Data Mining or Knowledge Discovery in Databases. This technology will be discussed later (Chapter 7).

References

AAMODT, A. and PLAZA, E., 1994, Cased-based reasoning – foundational issues, methodo-logical variations and system approaches, *AI Communications*, **7** (1), 39–59.
ALTHOFF, K.D., AURIOL, E., BARLETTA, R. and MANAGO, M., 1995, *A Review of Industrial Case-Based Reasoning Tools*, Oxford: AI Intelligence.
GOODALL, A., 1995, Preface in Althoff, K.D. *et al.*, *A Review of Industrial Case-Based Reasoning Tools*, Oxford: AI Intelligence.
HAMMOND, K.J., 1986, CHEF: A model of case-based planning, *Proceedings AAAI-86*, 267–271.
HAMMOND, K.J., 1989, *Case-Based Planning as a Memory Task*, London: Academic Press.
HENNESSY, D. and HINKLE, D., 1992, Applying case-based reasoning to autoclave loading, *IEEE Expert*, **7** (5), 21–26.

KEEN, M.J.R., 1993, Successful applications of case-based reasoning, *Manufacturing Intelligence*, **14**, 10–12.

KOLODNER, J., 1993, *Case-Based Reasoning*, San Mateo, CA: Morgan Kaufmann.

PERRAY, M., 1990, Comparative study between three knowledge acquisition techniques to build the same knowledge base: interview, induction and statistical analysis, *Proceedings of the 4th JIIA*, Paris.

QUINLAN, J.R., 1986, Induction of decision trees, *Machine Learning*, **1**, 81–106.

QUINLAN, J.R., 1993, *C4.5 Programs for Machine Learning*, San Mateo, CA: Morgan Kaufmann.

ROWE, R.C. and UPJOHN, N.G., 1993, An expert system for the identification and solution of film coating defects, *Pharm. Tech. Int.*, **5** (3), 34–38.

SHAW, F.J. and FIFER, R.A., 1988, *A Preliminary Report on Developing an Expert System for Computer-aided Formulation of Propellants*, Report No. BRL-TR-2895, Maryland: US Army Ballistic Research Laboratory.

5

Neural Networks, Genetic Algorithms and Fuzzy Logic

5.1 Introduction

The applications of artificial intelligence so far covered have all been restricted to sequential processing and only certain representations of knowledge and logic. A different approach involves using systems that mimic the processing capabilities of the human brain. The technology that attempts to achieve this is known as neural computing, artificial neural networks or more simply neural networks.

Research into neural networks started in the 1940s. The particular aspect that interested investigators was the powerful processing capabilities which emanated from the operation, in parallel, of very large numbers of relatively simple processing units known as neurons. However, research soon floundered due not only to the lack of adequate processing power of the computers of the day but also to inadequate mathematical models and it was not until the mid-1980s that improvements in both these areas led to a renaissance of neural network research. This chapter surveys the fundamentals of neural networks as well as dealing with two complementary technologies – genetic algorithms and fuzzy logic. The former is an attempt to optimise problem solving by imitating the evolutionary process by which biological systems self-organise and adapt; the latter an attempt to mimic the ability of the human mind to draw conclusions and generate responses based on vague, ambiguous, incomplete or imprecise information.

5.2 Neural Networks

Since the design of artificial neural networks has been inspired by the structure of the human brain, it is pertinent to briefly review the way it is believed to function. The fundamental processing unit of the brain is the neuron of which there are estimated to be in excess of 100 billion. The neurons are linked together by dendrites which serve to deliver messages to the neuron. Each neuron also has an output channel known as an axon by which signals can be transmitted unchanged or altered by synapses. These structures are able to increase or decrease the strength of the output signal and cause excitation or inhibition of a subsequent neuron.

Biological neuron

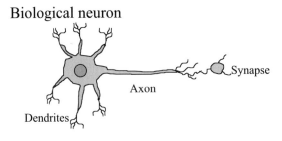

Artificial neuron

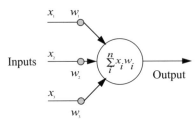

Comparison	
Biological	Artificial
Soma	Node
Dendrites	Inputs
Axon	Output
Synapse	Weight
Slow speed	Fast speed
Many Neurons - 10^9	Few Neurons - 10^2 - 10^3

Figure 5.1 A comparison between the biological and artificial neuron

In the artificial neural network the logic processing unit is the neuron which takes one or more inputs and produces an output. At each neuron every input has an associate weight that defines the relative importance of each input connected to the neuron. The neuron simply computes the weighted sum of all the inputs (the summation function) and calculates an output to be forwarded to another neuron. A comparison of both the biological and artificial neurons is shown in Figure 5.1.

Both biological and artificial neurons behave as threshold devices. The biological neuron is generally quiescent until the output voltage rises above a threshold value. Once this has been exceeded the neuron is switched on and the output signal is generated. In artificial neurons the threshold activation is computed by means of the transformation function (also known as the transfer or activation function).

The transformation function may be linear or non-linear, although the former will limit the neural network to implementation of simple linear functions e.g. addition and multiplication. Generally non-linear transformation functions are used allowing the neural network to implement more complex transformations and thus tackle a wider range of problems. Two types of transformation are shown in Figure 5.2.

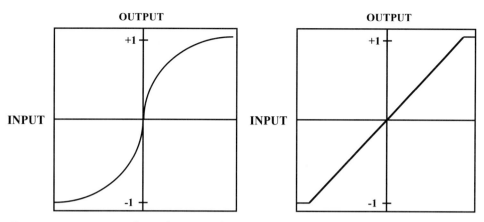

Figure 5.2   Two types of transformation function

The left hand plot is known as the sigmoid or logical activation function and is the preferred form for most types of neural network. The right hand plot is simpler to compute but can result in difficulties with training. The purpose of both transformations is to modify the output level of the neuron to a level between zero and one. The transformation is done before the output reaches the next neuron. Without such transformations the value of the output could be large and cause problems with computation in a network.

It can be seen from the above that neurons can only process numeric data. If a problem involves qualitative attributes then these must be pre-processed to numeric equivalents before they can be processed. An example of a neuron processing numeric data is shown in Figure 5.3. This simple processing unit is known as the elementary perceptron, an example of a feed forward system i.e. the transfer of data is in the forward direction only.

5.2.1   *Neural Network Architecture*

A neural network can consist of many hundreds of thousands of neurons. The method by which the neurons are organised is termed the network architecture. There are several that have been developed.

Multilayer perceptron (MLP) networks

The MLP network is one of the most popular and successful neural network architectures. It consists of identical neurons all interconnected and organised in layers with those in one layer connected to those in the next layer such that the outputs in one layer become the inputs in the subsequent layer. Data flow via the input layer, pass through one or more hidden layers and finally exit via the output layer. Hence it is known generically as a feed-forward network. Figure 5.4 illustrates the topology of a three layered MLP network with one hidden layer. Although, in theory, any number of hidden layers can be added, it has been found that for the majority of applications one hidden layer is sufficient. Multiple hidden layers are only of use for those systems with highly non-linear behaviour. In addition

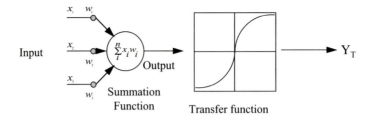

If inputs are $x_1 = 1$, $x_2 = 2$, $x_3 = 3$ and weights are $w_1 = 0.4$, $w_2 = 0.1$, $w_3 = 0.2$.

then Summation $S = \sum_i^n x_i w_i$

$$S = 1(0.4) + 2(0.1) + 3(0.2) = 1.2$$

If sigmoid transfer function used

i.e. $$Y_T = \frac{1}{1 + e^{-S}}$$

Then $$Y_T = \frac{1}{1 + e^{-1.2}} = 0.77$$

Figure 5.3 An example of an artificial neuron processing numeric data

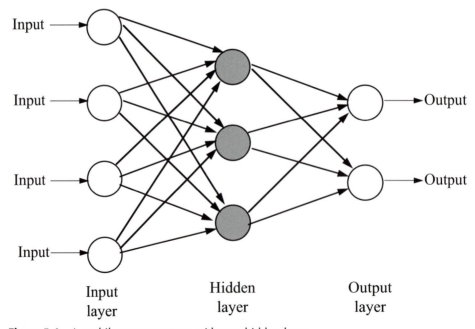

Figure 5.4 A multilayer perceptron with one hidden layer

multiple layers result in extended computation time and loss of processing speed. The number of neurons in the various layers should be kept as small as possible, consistent with the problem to be solved.

The MLP network is suitable for a wide range of applications including classification, pattern recognition, interpolation, prediction and process modelling. It is generally accepted that the performance of a well-designed MLP network is comparable with that achieved by classical statistical techniques. A full description of the MLP is given in Rummelhart and McClelland (1986).

Radial basis function (RBF) networks

The RBF network is a popular alternative to the MLP network to which it has a similar form in that it is a multilayer, feed-forward network. However, unlike the MLP network, the neurons in the hidden layer(s) are not identical to those in the input or output layers since they contain a statistical transformation based on a Gaussian function called the radial basis function. The size of the network is strongly dependent on the number of radial basis function neurons in the hidden layer.

The RBF network is suitable for a wide range of applications including classification, pattern recognition, interpolation and process modelling. It can model local data more accurately, it has a greater non-linear capability than the MLP network and it is easier to train. However, it is not as well suited for applications with a large number of inputs and there is no generally accepted method for setting the radial basis functions for each neuron.

A special type of the RBF network is the Gaussian functional link network which uses the transformation distributed over the input space as additional processing neurons in the input layer of the network. It is a specific architecture to CAD/ Chem (Chapter 6).

Learning vector quantisation (LVQ) networks

The LVQ network is a feed-forward network similar to the MLP network. Because it provides discrete rather than continuous outputs, it is really only suitable for classification applications. In practice these networks are useful when there is an imbalance in the number of examples from each class and where individual classes have a rich variety of forms.

Recurrent neural networks

In contrast to other neural network architectures, the recurrent neural network employs feedback and hence can be considered to have a form of memory. In this network, outputs from the output layer are fed back to a set of input neurons (Figure 5.5). Hence the recurrent neural network contains five layers: an input and an output with a set of three hidden layers – one containing the previous input, another corresponding to the previous output state and the third containing the output vector corresponding to the current prediction.

These networks are very useful for storing information about time and are particularly suitable for time series prediction. However, in problems where prediction depends both on the time series and related information the MLP network will perform better.

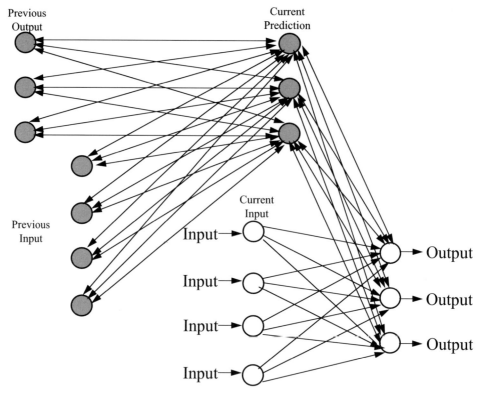

Figure 5.5   A recurrent neural network

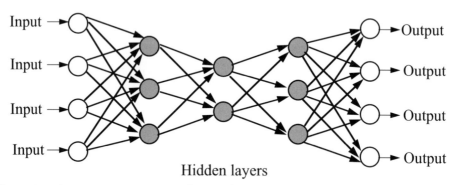

Figure 5.6   An auto-associative neural network

Auto-associative neural networks

The auto-associative neural network is a special form of the MLP network and consists of two MLP networks connected back to back with a common middle layer (Figure 5.6). A feature of this architecture is that the number of neurons in the hidden layers must be less than the number in the input and output layers otherwise the network would simply copy the inputs through to the outputs. This feature forces the neural network to learn relationships in the input data. Hence these networks are ideal for data validation.

Functional link neural (FLN) networks

These are feed-forward networks which use a variety of transformations based on linear and trigonometric functions which can increase the number of neurons in either the input or hidden layers. The role of the functional link transformations is not to introduce new information but to enhance the existing data. These enhancements are often used in the input layer and can result in a network with a simpler structure and no hidden layers. If used with neurons in the hidden layers of an MLP network, the enhancements can be useful for complex systems with non-linear behaviour. Several enhancements are present in the neural network architectures provided by CAD/Chem (Chapter 6).

Kohonen networks

These networks, also known as self-organising maps, have a single layer of neurons. During training, clustering of these neurons based on similarity functions occurs producing a feature map as an output. The feature map may have more than two dimensions depending on the problem. The Kohonen network is particularly useful in applications where there are a large number of examples and there is a need to identify groups with different features. They are also effective in applications where there is an imbalance in the number of examples from the different groups that need to be identified. The Kohonen network does not need labelled training data and can be used when little is known about the data.

5.2.2 Training Neural Networks

Unlike conventional computer programs which are explicitly programmed, neural networks are trained with previous examples (the training set). Training (sometimes referred to as learning) can either be supervised or unsupervised or a hybrid dependent on the network architecture (Table 5.1).

Supervised training is the process by which the network is presented with a series of matching input and output examples and the weights of the neurons are adjusted such that the output for a specific input is close to the desired output. The difference between actual and desired outputs is usually quantified by means of an error function not dissimilar to those used in statistics.

Table 5.1 Training processes for neural networks

Architecture	Training process
Multilayer perceptron	Supervised
Radial basis function	Supervised
Functional link	Supervised
Learning vector quantisation	Supervised
Recurrent	Supervised
Auto-associative	Supervised
Kohonen	Unsupervised
Gaussian functional link	Hybrid

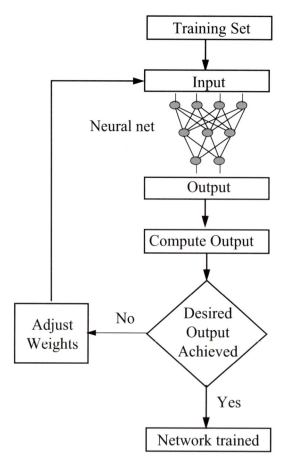

Figure 5.7 The process used for neural network training

The training process is an iterative one (Figure 5.7) whereby the error function at each forward pass is calculated and then passed backward through the network. Each pass through a training set is known as an epoch and the algorithm used to compute the errors is known as a training algorithm. There are several training algorithms available for the supervised training of MLP, auto-associative and recurrent networks, all based on the back-propagation of error technique.

The most commonly used method is the gradient descent with momentum or standard back-propagation algorithm also known as the generalised delta rule. This calculates the direction in n dimensions (n being the number of weights to be adjusted) of the weight changes that would cause the greatest reduction in the error function. The amount of adjustment per pass is controlled by the momentum, which is a proportion of the previously calculated weight change, and the learning rate a multiplication factor used to determine the magnitude of successive weight changes. If the learning rate is too high, the weights will have too high an adjustment at each epoch with the result that there is no convergence between the output and the desired output. However, if the learning rate is too low training time becomes excessively long. Establishing these is generally done by experimentation during training. There are many refinements to this algorithm designed to improve training.

A second series of algorithms used for these networks includes the Line Search algorithms which compute a descent direction and perform a line minimisation in that direction. Once a minimum has been found a new direction is computed. A well known example of this group of algorithms is the Conjugate Gradient algorithm.

Specific training algorithms are available for the Learning Vector Quantisation networks while the Radial Basis Function networks require two stages to training: the selection of values for the radial basis functions followed by the setting of the output layer weights. Details of these algorithms are given in the DTI *Best Practice Guidelines for Developing Neural Computing Applications* (1994) and other textbooks.

Unsupervised training, used specifically for the Kohonen network, is the process by which the network is presented with the input data alone and the weights adjusted such that similar inputs consistently result in the same output i.e. the network learns to recognise patterns in the input data. The training algorithms for this type of training are designed to produce clusters of similar input data and place similar clusters close together in an output map. Details on these algorithms are given in Kohonen (1990). Clustering is a very useful data analysis tool in its own right highlighting patterns in data which may not have been obvious. Clustering large data sets often results in the production of distinct subsets which can then be more accurately modelled using supervised training.

A problem specific to neural networks is that of overtraining i.e. the network performs well on the training data set but poorly on the unseen test data set. This is because the network starts to learn the noise in the training set due to it being too complex. Figure 5.8 illustrates how complexity affects the test results. It should be noted that complexity involves more than just the number of neurons and hidden layers (i.e. the size of the network) but also includes the constraints on the weight values. Overtraining is an important factor in the design and optimisation of neural networks, the ideal network being one that has a complexity commensurate with good performance on unseen test data. There are no hard and fast rules for achieving the optimum compromise; it can only be done by trial and error.

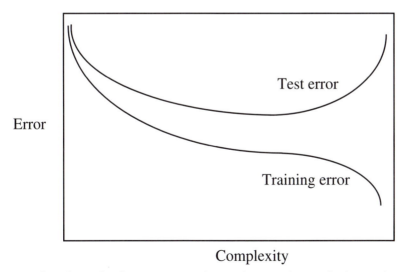

Figure 5.8   The relationship between network complexity and error displaying the concept of overtraining

For full descriptions of neural network architectures and training algorithms see Wasserman (1989), Alexander and Morton (1990), Beale and Jackson (1990), Hertz *et al.* (1991), Davalo and Naim (1991), Freeman and Skapura (1991) and Nelson and Illingworth (1991). For an excellent introduction to building neural networks the reader is referred to Skapura's textbook of the same title (Skapura, 1996).

5.2.3 *Advantages of Neural Networks*

Although neural networks may never approach the ability of the human brain they have a number of attributes which can be used with advantage in a wide number of applications:

- Diversity – neural networks are able to deal with complex, real world applications where data is fuzzy (i.e. uncertain and incomplete) and non-linear. This is in contrast to other processing techniques which are based on assumptions about linearity. Neural networks are able to deal with subjective descriptions such as 'fast' or 'slow' or 'hard' or 'soft' provided that the user can define numerically what each of the terms mean.

- Ability to learn – neural networks operate by discovering new relationships within the input data. Hence they are particularly suited to problems where rules are difficult to develop or the solution is complex and difficult to specify but where there is an abundance of data.

- Ability to generalise – once trained a neural network can deal with unseen data and generate correct responses.

- Ability to deal with incomplete or noisy data – neural networks are able to extract information from incomplete data. Because they are essentially statistical systems they are able to recognise underlying noise.

- Fault tolerance – since there are many processing neurons in a neural network, damage to a few does not bring the system to a halt.

- Speed and efficiency – although training a neural network can be relatively slow and demanding of computer power, once trained neural networks are inherently fast. This is because they consist of a large number of interconnected processing units all operating in parallel.

- Flexibility and maintenance – neural networks are very flexible in the way they can adapt to new and changing environments. They are relatively easy to maintain.

5.2.4 *Development Tools*

Like any other application of AI, neural networks can be programmed with a programming language, a development tool or both. Since a major portion of programming deals with the training algorithms, the transfer and the summation functions, it makes sense to use development tools in which these features are pre-programmed. A number of commercial tools are now available (Table 5.2) but as with any other development tools their use will always be constrained by the facilities they provide. Important factors to be considered are:

Table 5.2 Some representative examples of neural network development tools and their suppliers

Tool	Supplier
AIM	AbTech Corp.
BrainMaker	California Scientific Software
Braincel	Promised Land Technologies
CAD/Chem	AI Ware Inc.
DANA	Neural Ware Inc.
Genesis	Neural Systems Inc.
N-Net	AI Ware Inc.
Neuro Shell	Ward Systems Inc.
Neuro Windows	Ward Systems Inc.
NeuDesk	Neural Computer Services Ltd
Neural Works Professional	Neural Ware Inc.
Win Brain	Applied Cognetics Inc.

- Modular structure allowing integration to non-neural network modules e.g. spreadsheets, databases.
- Adequate facilities for importing and exporting data.
- Facilities for pre-processing and post-processing data.
- Support for a library of neural network architectures.
- Assistance in the choice of the appropriate neural network.
- Facilities for network editing i.e. changing the number of neurons/hidden layers.
- Selection of end training algorithm criteria.
- Selection of training algorithm, to suit network architecture.
- Facilities for analysing the performance of the network.
- Facilities for producing source code which can run on a dedicated deliverable system.

Of all the development tools listed in Table 5.2 only one, CAD/Chem from AI Ware Inc., has been specifically designed for product formulators to develop neural networks to model formulations. Its functionality will be discussed in Chapter 6.

In the product formulation domain several tools have been used to develop neural networks to model formulations viz. CAD/Chem for adhesives, paints (Gill and Shutt, 1992; VerDuin, 1994) and pharmaceutical tablets (Colbourn and Rowe, 1996); Neural Works Professional for sustained release tablets (Hussain *et al.*, 1994) and DANA (Design Advisor/Neural Analyser) for directly compressed tablets (Turkoglu *et al.*, 1995). All these applications will be discussed in detail in Chapter 10.

5.2.5 *Comparison with Expert Systems*

Neural networks have been labelled by some as sixth generation computing, leading to the erroneous impression that they will replace fifth generation computing, expert systems. In fact the two technologies have complimentary characteristics as

Table 5.3 A comparison of neural networks and expert systems

Neural networks	Expert systems
Primarily numeric approach	Primarily symbolic approach
Associative (inductive) reasoning	Logical (declarative) reasoning
Parallel processing	Sequential processing
Driven by data	Driven by knowledge
Little domain knowledge	High domain knowledge
Short development time	Long development time
Suited for pattern recognition	Poor in pattern recognition
No explanation facilities	Explanation available
Adaptive and flexible	Little flexibility
Fault tolerant	Not fault tolerant

summarised in Table 5.3 and in many instances the two technologies are not in competition. Neural networks can be used in situations where rules are extremely difficult to develop but where there is a large amount of historical data. In these cases neural networks can be used to identify clusters and patterns that may subsequently lead to the generation of rules for expert systems. In fact neural networks are now recognised as a learning technology fundamental to the success of Data Mining and Knowledge Discovery in Databases (Chapter 7).

5.3 Genetic Algorithms

As can be seen from the previous discussion neural networks are ideal for modelling complex systems with non-linear behaviour. Once a model has been produced it is easy to predict the outcome of any change in the input parameters i.e. it is easy to pose 'what if' questions and obtain accurate responses (Figure 5.9). This consultation mode can then be used to provide insight into the problem. However, attempting to discover the combination of input parameters that will provide an

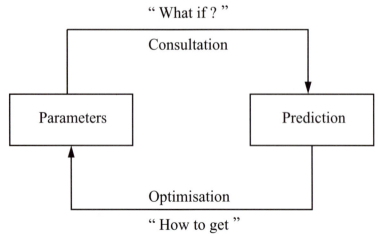

Figure 5.9 The relationship between consultation and optimisation

optimum result using consultation is, at worst, a tedious and time consuming task and, at best, a matter of luck. A way to search the model space to such a combination of input parameters is by the use of genetic algorithms.

Two definitions of a genetic algorithm that are useful in describing its function are:

'The genetic algorithm is an optimisation technique based on evolutionary principles' (Cartwright, 1993).

'A software program that learns from experience in a similar (simplified) manner to the way in which biological systems learn' (Turban, 1995).

In essence the genetic algorithm is loosely based on the biological principles of genetic variation and natural selection mimicking the basic ideas of evolution over many generations. It works with a population of individuals each of which is a candidate solution to the problem. These individuals then reproduce through mating or mutation, all the time evolving new solutions to the problem. Ultimately after several generations an optimum solution will be found.

5.3.1   *Structure*

Although the genetic algorithm is based on the concepts of biological evolution each individual in a genetic algorithm population exists in the form of a string or ordered sequence of numbers representing a numerical solution to the problem (e.g., 20, 45, 43, 65, 22, 34) and the mechanism of operation is based on logic and mathematics. For a genetic algorithm to function it must possess several features:

- A numerical description of how good any solution is to the problem. This is generally referred to as the fitness function and can be any arbitrary relationship that gives a high value if the solution is judged a good one and a low value if the solution is judged a bad one. Often the relationship is defined in such a way as to accentuate the difference between good and bad solutions.

- A logical method of selecting individual solutions to become parents of the next generation of solutions. In some cases this can simply be accomplished by selection based on the highest fitness functions. However as is known through evolution, survival of the fittest only provides guidelines by which to construct the next generation. It is not completely deterministic since sometimes poorly adapted individuals may manage to produce good offspring and well adapted individuals may produce poor offspring. To accommodate these concepts, genetic algorithms use a biased random-selection methodology, i.e. parents are randomly selected in such a way that the 'best' attributes/strings in the population have the greatest chance of being selected.

- A logical method of mixing the various elements of the strings within an individual to produce a new solution. This process, analogous to the mixing of genes that accompanies reproduction and mutation of chromosomes, is performed by the genetic algorithm using crossover and mutation operators. Crossover operators may be of a variety of forms including cyclic, order based and position based. They involve swapping parts of the string of a parent with the corresponding part of the other with the result that two further individuals are

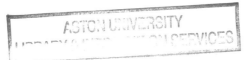

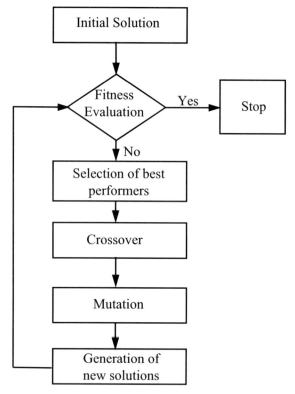

Figure 5.10   The genetic algorithm cycle

produced. Mutation operators may also have a variety of forms including displacement mutation, insertion mutation, inversion mutation or exchange mutation. They involve the random selection of individual elements or groups of elements within a string and their insertion back in a different position or different order. The individuals so formed are then added to the population to produce an extended population which may then be reduced to its original size by some selection procedure.

A diagrammatic form of the genetic algorithm cycle is shown in Figure 5.10. Output from each cycle or generation is in the form of either tables or more commonly graphs of the type shown in Figure 5.11. Typically, after a few generations most of the individuals tend to be clustered around the maximum fitness function. As the number of generations increases the overall fitness of the population as indicated by the average population fitness increases until convergence is reached (Figure 5.12).

While it may appear, at first sight, to be a random search of the model space, the improvement seen in Figure 5.12 does indicate that the algorithm provides an effective directed search technique. The reason for this is due to the schema theorem (describing the rate that good solutions or schema proliferate) or the fundamental theorem of genetic algorithms which can be described mathematically to give a general equation (Goldberg, 1989; Cartwright, 1993).

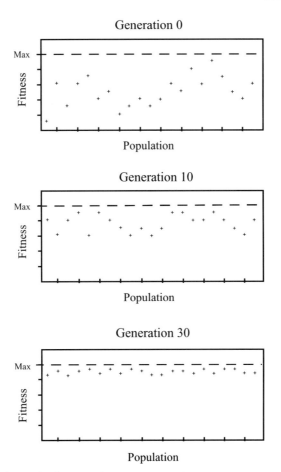

Figure 5.11 The change in fitness values per generation

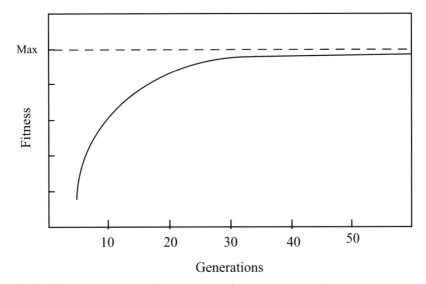

Figure 5.12 The change in population average fitness per generation

5.3.2 *Advantages*

The genetic algorithm is an effective optimisation technique for several reasons:

- It is a stochastic algorithm, not a deterministic one, i.e. it relies on random elements in parts of its operation rather than being determined by specific rules (cf. Rapson–Newton method which is a hill-climbing gradient/derivative method). Hence it is very effective for optimising systems where there are multiple maxima or significant noise.
- It investigates many possible solutions simultaneously, each investigation learning about a different region. The effect of the collective memory and the ability of solutions to communicate with each other make the algorithm very effective at finding global maxima.
- It requires no additional information about the problem.
- It is not susceptible to the initial starting point of the search. Deterministic methods can get trapped into solutions other than the global minima/maxima because they are based on steepest ascent methods and therefore are prone to the initial starting point.

For a genetic algorithm to work effectively it requires a rapid feedback of fitness values. Hence the combination of a genetic algorithm with a neural network is ideal. Such a combination is shown in Figure 5.13 and is the concept used by CAD/Chem from AI Ware Inc., where a formulation is modelled using a neural network and then optimised using a genetic algorithm (Chapter 6). Such a process has been

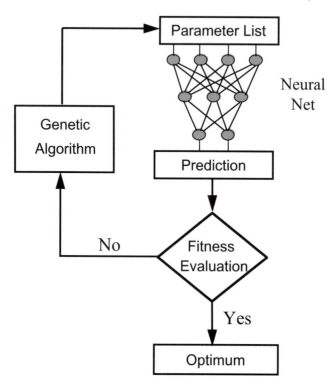

Figure 5.13 The relationship between neural networks and a genetic algorithm as used in the optimisation of a model

used to optimise formulations for adhesives and paints (Gill and Shutt, 1992; VerDuin, 1994) and pharmaceutical tablets (Colbourn and Rowe, 1996).

5.4 Fuzzy Logic

Fuzzy logic is a powerful problem solving technique with applications in control and decision making. It derives its power from its ability to draw conclusions and generate responses based on vague, ambiguous, incomplete and imprecise information. To simulate this process of human reasoning it applies the mathematical theory of fuzzy sets first defined in the 1960s by Professor Lofti Zadeh. Zadeh extended the traditional definition of a logic premise from having just two extremes (either completely true or completely false) to one in which there is a range in degree of truth from 0 to 100 per cent i.e. there is a range from partially true to partially false (Zadeh, 1965). Fuzzy logic thus extends traditional logic in two ways: first, sets can be labelled qualitatively using linguistic terms (e.g., hot, cold, warm); and second, the elements of these sets can be assigned varying degrees of membership called membership functions.

Figure 5.14 shows diagrammatically fuzzy sets for temperature. The *x* axis is temperature with ranges for the fuzzy sets cold, cool, warm and hot. The *y* axis represents the membership function and ranges 0 to 100. It can be seen that the temperature 16°C can be regarded as both cool and warm with membership functions of 80 and 20 respectively. In other words 16°C is cool to a greater degree than it is warm. The membership function is very subjective in nature and is a matter of definition rather than measurement. Another way of looking at it is to view the *y* axis as possibility values. For a very readable account of fuzziness and fuzzy logic the reader is referred to McNeill and Freiberger (1993) and Partridge and Hussain (1994).

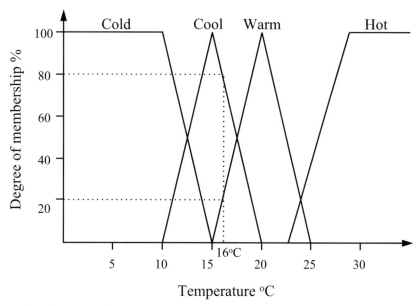

Figure 5.14 Fuzzy sets for temperature

From Figure 5.14 it can be seen that overlapping between set boundaries is desirable (an overlap of 25 per cent between adjacent fuzzy sets is a general rule of thumb (Viot, 1993)). This process permits the interaction between linguistic terms (cold, cool, warm and hot) and the membership functions making the terms meaningful to a computer. As a result a developer can express or modify the behaviour of a system using natural language enhancing the possibility of concise description of complex tasks.

5.4.1 Applications

The flow of data through a fuzzy expert system is shown in Figure 5.15. Implementation is via three transformations: first, a fuzzification process that uses predefined membership functions to map each system input into one or more degrees of membership; second, a rule evaluation stage where rules are evaluated by combining degrees of membership to produce output strengths; and third, a defuzzification process that computes the system outputs based on the output strengths and output membership functions. The last stage is necessary to decipher the meaning of the vague fuzzy actions and resolve conflicts between competing actions.

Fuzzy logic is difficult to apply where there are problems with supplying definitions for membership functions but it is ideal where input data is provided by

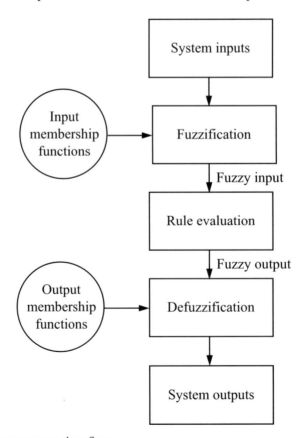

Figure 5.15   Fuzzy system data flow

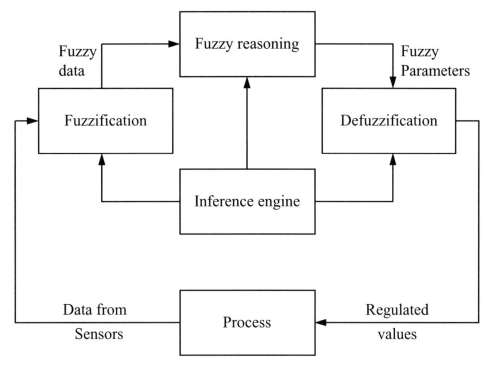

Figure 5.16 A fuzzy logic controller

sensors. Hence fuzzy logic is used extensively in the area of control (Rouvray, 1997). A diagram of a fuzzy logic controller is shown in Figure 5.16. Such systems are used in regulating automatic braking systems in cars, autofocusing in cameras, controlling the oxygen in cement kilns and many others (Turban, 1995). Fuzzy logic is also used in business applications for evaluating applications for loans, purchasing and selling stocks and shares, and in medical diagnosis. It is also interesting to note that fuzzy logic is also used in CAD/Chem from AI Ware Inc. for modelling product formulations (Chapter 6) where it is used to specify preferences in product properties before optimisation. The desirability functions used are, in effect, fuzzy logic membership functions (VerDuin, 1995).

Fuzzy logic can also be combined with neural networks to produce neuro-fuzzy techniques. These combine the generality and flexibility of representation, a feature of fuzzy logic, with the powerful learning and adaptive capability of neural networks (Jang *et al.*, 1997). Fuzzy networks are neural-processing structures that emulate the fuzzy logic functions. They are similar in architecture to the multilayer perceptron but are not adaptive; each must be constructed specifically for its intended application (Skapura, 1996). The multilayer perceptron network can also be used to mimic the process of fuzzy inference, the only significant difference being how each processing element is interconnected between layers. In the multilayer perceptron each element is completely interconnected between layers with each connection being a specific weight. In the fuzzy inference network, however, connections are only between elements that require them for specific rules and there are no associated weights (Skapura, 1996).

Table 5.4 Some representative examples of fuzzy logic tools and their suppliers

Tool	Supplier
Fuzzy Inference Development Environment (FIDE)	Aptronics Inc.
Fuzzy Control Package	Byotronic Int. Ltd
FuziCalc	FuzziWare Inc.
Fuzzy Knowledge Builder	Fuzzy System Engineering
CubiCalc	HyperLogic Corp.
TILGEN, TILShell	Togai InfraLogic Inc.
Neufuzzy	NCS Manufacturing Intelligence

5.4.2 *Advantages and Tools*

Fuzzy logic has many advantages:

- It has a wide applicability especially to problems too awkward to solve with conventional technology.
- It provides flexibility allowing the consideration of all possibilities including the unexpected.
- It is forgiving in that high accuracy of input is not a prerequisite.
- It does not require mathematical modelling of the domain.
- It allows for non-linear behaviour.
- It is easy to implement, reducing development times and increasing system maintainability.

Fuzzy logic is easy to implement using standard code in C. However fuzzy development tools exist which allow the developer to focus more on the application. Some representative examples of fuzzy logic tools are given in Table 5.4.

5.5 Conclusion

Neural networks, genetic algorithms and fuzzy logic are rapidly expanding technologies finding many applications not least in the domain of product formulation (Chapters 6 and 9). In addition all three technologies can be applied to Knowledge Discovery in Databases (KDD) and Data Mining and are present in several Data Mining tools (Chapter 7).

References

ALEXANDER, I. and MORTON, H., 1990, *An Introduction to Neural Computing*, London: Chapman and Hall.

BEALE, R. and JACKSON, T., 1990, *Neural Computing – An Introduction*, Bristol: IOP Publishing.

CARTWRIGHT, H.M., 1993, *Applications of Artificial Intelligence in Chemistry*, Oxford: Oxford University Press.

COLBOURN, E.A. and ROWE, R.C., 1996, Modelling and optimisation of a tablet formulation using neural networks and genetic algorithms, *Pharm. Tech. Eur.*, **8** (9), 46–55.

DAVALO, E. and NAIM, P., 1991, *Neural Networks*, London: Macmillan Education.

DTI, 1994, *Best Practice Guidelines for Developing Neural Computing Applications*, London: DTI.

FREEMAN, J.A. and SKAPURA, D.M., 1991, *Neural Network Algorithms, Applications and Programming Techniques*, Houston: Addison-Wesley.

GILL, T. and SHUTT, J., 1992, Optimising product formulations using neural networks, *Scientific Computing and Automation*, **5** (9), 18–26.

GOLDBERG, D.E., 1989, *Genetic Algorithms in Search, Optimisation and Machine Learning*, Reading, MA: Addison-Wesley.

HERTZ, J., KROGH, A. and PALMER, R., 1991, *Introduction to the Theory of Neural Computing*, Reading, MA: Addison-Wesley.

HUSSAIN, A.S., SHIVANAND, P. and JOHNSON, R.D., 1994, Application of neural computing in pharmaceutical product development: computer aided formulation design, *Drug Dev. Ind. Pharm.*, **20**, 1739–1752.

JANG, J.S.R., SUN, C.T. and MIZUTANI, E., 1997, *Neuro-Fuzzy and Soft Computing*, Englewood Cliffs, NJ: Prentice-Hall.

KOHONEN, T., 1990, The self-organising map, *Proc. IEEE*, **78**, 1464–1480.

MCNEILL, D. and FREIBERGER, P., 1993, *Fuzzy Logic*, New York: Simon and Schuster.

NELSON, M.M. and ILLINGWORTH, W.T., 1991, *A Practical Guide to Neural Networks*, Reading, MA: Addison-Wesley.

PARTRIDGE, D. and HUSSAIN, K.M., 1994, *Knowledge-Based Information Systems*, London: McGraw-Hill.

ROUVRAY, D.H., 1997, Fuzzy logic: a new tool for chemical process control, *Chem. Ind.*, No. 2, 60–62.

RUMMELHART, D.E. and MCCLELLAND, J.L., 1986, *Parallel distributed processing: explorations in the microstructure of cognition*, Cambridge, MA: MIT Press.

SKAPURA, D.M., 1996, *Building Neural Networks*, Reading, MA: Addison-Wesley.

TURBAN, E., 1995, *Decision Support Systems and Expert Systems*, 4th edition, Englewood Cliffs, NJ: Prentice-Hall.

TURKOGLU, M., OZARSLAN, R. and SAKR, A., 1995, Artificial neural network analysis of a direct compression tabletting study, *Eur. J. Pharm. Biopharm.*, **41**, 315–322.

VERDUIN, W.H., 1994, Knowledge-based systems for formulation optimisation, *Tappi Journal*, **77** (8), 100–104.

VERDUIN, W.H., 1995, *Better Products Faster*, New York: Irwin.

VIOT, G., 1993, Fuzzy logic in C, *Dr Dobb's Journal*, **18** (2), 40–49.

WASSERMAN, P.D., 1989, *Neural Computing Theory and Practice*, New York: Van Nostrand Reinhold.

ZADEH, L.A., 1965, Fuzzy sets, *Information and Control*, **8** (3), 338–353.

6

The CAD/Chem Formulation Design and Optimisation Program

E.A. COLBOURN
Oxford Materials Ltd

6.1 Introduction

A general overview of neural networks and genetic algorithms has been presented in Chapter 5. These technologies have been incorporated into CAD/Chem, a Windows-based computer package developed by AI Ware Inc. of Cleveland, Ohio, specifically to address the needs of product formulators. Within CAD/Chem neural networks are used to generate models which link inputs and outputs, and genetic algorithms are employed for efficient optimisation in the multidimensional design space. The current chapter discusses the capabilities of CAD/Chem and its relevance to product formulation. In order to illustrate in more detail how a program like CAD/Chem can be applied in product design and optimisation, a specific example of tablet formulation will be used throughout the chapter. This example will be discussed again in Chapter 10; it is based on published data from Kesavan and Peck (1995) and the application of CAD/Chem to this problem has been previously reported by Colbourn and Rowe (1996).

Like all packages based on neural networks, CAD/Chem is data driven. This means that it relies on experimental results provided by the user and, in order to develop a useful model, these must cover both sides of a cause and effect relationship. CAD/Chem has the usual advantages conferred by neural networks in that it can deal with historical data, incomplete and fuzzy results and non-linear problems. These make it especially attractive for complex formulations and for improving formulations which may have evolved over time with the addition of new ingredients. The incorporation of optimisation into the same package allows users both to carry out 'what if' changes in formulation and also to optimise to find which ingredients will give their desired properties, all using the same model. This is illustrated in Figure 6.1.

Since CAD/Chem is designed to be used by product formulators rather than by neural network experts it is essential that its complex technologies be easy to use. Integration of 2D and 3D graphics, a fully Windows-compatible interface using terminology familiar to formulators, and extensive on-line help and tips accessible within the program all assist to make this possible.

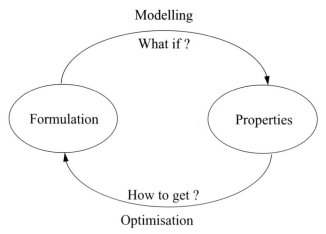

Figure 6.1   Using the same model for 'what if' experiments and optimisation

6.2   **Information Flow**

CAD/Chem has three main modes of operation, which involve loading data, developing the model and using the model. For a new problem these are carried out sequentially and the user is automatically moved on to the next phase once the current one is completed. At each stage the results are stored to a separate sub-directory on the hard disk. This means that the information is readily accessible during subsequent sessions.

Once the model is available, it is possible at any stage to return to it using CAD/Chem in the 'consult' mode either for 'what if' experiments or for optimisation. Most users find this is their preferred way of working and tend to use the program every fortnight or so for a design session which will guide their next phase of experiments.

It is also possible to re-enter the program at earlier stages. For example, one can use the original data, once loaded, to develop a variety of models by re-entering the training phase. Each model can be saved so that comparison between models is straightforward. Finally, new data can be added, for example, if further experimentation has been undertaken a new model can be developed taking account of these new results.

Thus, there are three possible entry points into CAD/Chem depending on what prior modelling work has been undertaken with the software. This is illustrated in Figure 6.2.

6.3   **Data**

As with most computer programs it is necessary to load data. In the case of CAD/Chem, the data are inputs (ingredients and process conditions) and properties (measured experimentally) organised into records, each of which corresponds to a single experiment. The inputs and outputs are jointly referred to as variables and CAD/Chem imposes no inherent limit on the number of variables which can be treated; the number is limited only by the memory available within the computer.

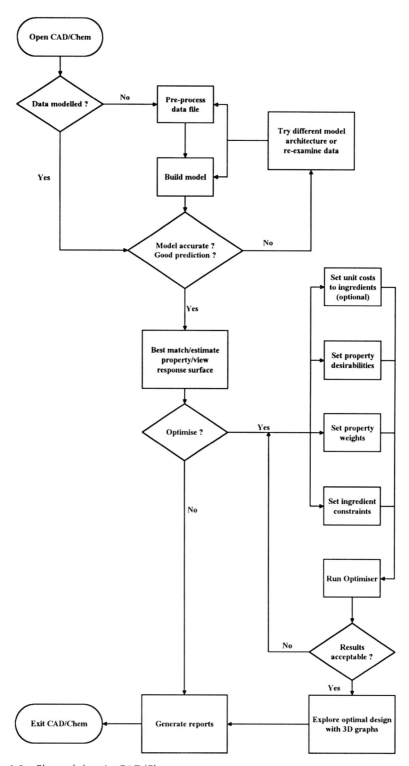

Figure 6.2 Flow of data in CAD/Chem

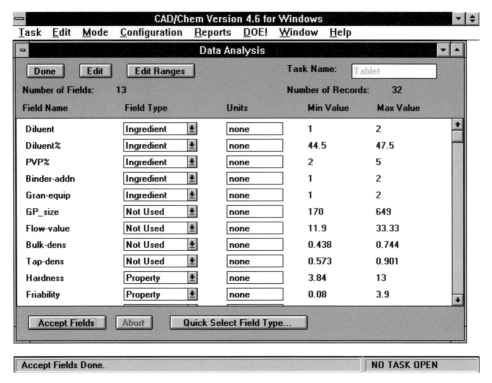

Figure 6.3 The Load Data workscreen, with variables marked as Ingredients, Properties or Not Used

Similarly, there is no limit on the number of data records which can be used, although for large problems, training times will be longer.

If data are available within a standard spreadsheet they can be transferred into the CAD/Chem input screen by a simple cut and paste using the Windows clipboard. Each record should be saved as a single line in the spreadsheet using only numerical values for the variables. The exception to the 'all numerical' rule is the first line of the spreadsheet, which contains the variable names specified by the user. These names will be used throughout CAD/Chem for the current formulation problem and the use of relevant ingredient and property names gives an instant familiarity to the user. Within the spreadsheet there must be no empty cells or data will not be loaded correctly. The treatment of missing data is discussed later.

Each spreadsheet file within CAD/Chem is limited to 500 records – usually more than adequate for most formulation problems. If more data records are available they can be incorporated into other CAD/Chem spreadsheets during the data loading phase. At the end of the data loading CAD/Chem will merge them into the same datafile so that they will all be treated together during the training phase.

In CAD/Chem it is necessary for the user to specify which of the variables are inputs and which are outputs, so that they will be handled correctly. This information is supplied during the stage of loading the data into the program using simple pull-down menus. There are three options for each variable – Ingredient, Property and Not Used. Although Not Used would seem at first sight to be unimportant it can be useful in, for example, seeing whether a different model is developed if a specific variable is omitted. Figure 6.3 shows the tablet formulation example, developing a model which goes straight from the initial formulation to tablet properties, leaving the granule properties as Not Used.

There is an optional ability to specify the units in which the variables are measured. This can be a useful reminder if the formulator returns to the problem months or years after the initial model development was undertaken or if datasets are shared between different researchers.

6.3.1 *Quality and Quantity*

One of the first questions which arises in using a neural network package usually concerns how many data records are required. It is generally believed that neural networks are data-hungry and that good models will only be developed when there are very many more data records (experiments) than there are inputs. However, experience on a wide variety of formulation problems has shown that, in general, adequate models can be developed when there are only three to four times as many experiments as there are input properties. If there are about ten times as many experiments as inputs, very good models incorporating subtleties in the cause and effect relationships can be developed. Although Design of Experiments (sometimes known as Statistical Experimental Design) is gaining wider use in research, frequently companies have a considerable quantity of historic data representing years of effort. Neural networks cope very well with the random nature of most historical data.

Data must be in numerical form to be treated by the neural network. This does not preclude the possibility of properties being logical items like 'true/false', or qualitative measures like 'good, indifferent, bad', but in such cases a numerical scale like 0/1, or 1/2/3, must be assigned. Neural networks can also handle missing data if, for example, a particular input or output has not been measured. In the case of CAD/Chem, the numerical value -99999 is used to flag missing data. Note that 0 (zero) would not be a suitable flag since it can be a valid value for the amount of an ingredient present. Missing inputs are treated by 'clustering' the data; the missing value is taken to be the centroid of the relevant cluster, however the user has the opportunity to replace this with his or her own value using the inbuilt data-editing facilities. Missing outputs are usually handled by leaving that particular experimental record out of the model; by default, the neural network develops a model for each property (the so-called Independent Outputs mode) so the experiment is only omitted for the model developed for that one property.

The data record can also be qualified with a 'belief' factor if there is a suspicion that it may not be completely reliable. If, for example, something happens during an experiment which causes the researcher to question the validity of the measurements, the experimental record could still be included in the model but be given a reduced weighting which reflects the formulator's view of the degree of uncertainty. A belief factor of 1 is taken by default since experiments are assumed to be wholly reliable. A belief factor of 0 would mean that the result was completely unreliable and would not be used in developing the model.

Within the data loading phase there is an automatic check to see if any input (ingredient or process variable) values are held constant. If there are, a warning message is displayed asking if the user wishes to exclude it from data training.

Since there is no information on the variation of this particular input this is a sensible course to take.

6.3.2   *Data Preprocessing*

Various types of data processing can be undertaken prior to training the neural network. First, CAD/Chem incorporates graphical techniques which allow the results to be examined for outliers and to ensure that there is an adequate coverage of the design space. Second, a Statistics button on the data spreadsheet allows the user to determine whether there are correlations between the data and to look at the minimum, maximum and mean values, examining the variance and standard deviation in the data.

For complex data sets data clustering might be a sensible first step. CAD/Chem carries out the data clustering by calculating the Euclidean distance between two points in the multidimensional space and determining whether they are within a user-defined cut-off distance. If so, they are included as part of the same cluster and the cluster is represented by its centroid. This clustering technique is used to provide values for missing inputs as discussed previously. It can also be used to resolve 'conflicting records' i.e. records where the inputs are the same but the outputs are different. Such conflicts can arise if, for example, an experiment is performed more than once to get a measure of the experimental variation. Data clustering can also be used when there are a lot of experimental records to reduce very large problems to a manageable size. However this is not typically the case in formulation problems and is more likely to be relevant for process applications.

One further aspect of preprocessing may be necessary. Data are put into CAD/Chem as numbers which can have any magnitude. This is obviously very convenient for the user since minimal preprocessing is needed and the results are displayed in an immediately recognisable form. However, the neural network requires that the variables be normalised prior to training and so will scale them accordingly. If the user plans to explore 'what if' possibilities which lie outside the training set, the data range should be adjusted during the data loading phase so that the expected endpoints are used for the normalisation. This increases the reliability of the extrapolation outside the training data set. To facilitate the procedure an Edit Ranges button is provided, which gives the user access to a workscreen in which the new endpoints can be readily entered.

6.3.3   *The Tablet Formulation Data Set*

The data used in the tablet formulation problem are those published by Kesavan and Peck (1995). There are 32 reported experiments, with the possibility of varying the amount of two different diluents (lactose or dicalcium phosphate dihydrate) and of using two different granulating techniques, fluidised bed or high shear granulation. The amount of polyvinylpyrrolidone, used as a binder, is allowed to vary and can be added either wet or dry. The model drug, caffeine, is kept in the same amount (by weight) in each formulation as is the amount of corn starch (used as a disintegrant) and magnesium stearate (which functions as a lubricant to facilitate tablet ejection from the die). Properties measured are those of the granules (mean granule size, flow value, bulk density and tap density) and of the final tablets (hardness, friability, thickness and disintegration time). The data input for this problem are shown in Figure 6.3. In setting up the data set, the granulation equipment and the diluent type and binder addition are all set using integer flags. Thus in Figure 6.3, for the diluents, 1 refers to lactose and 2 refers to dicalcium phosphate dihydrate; for the granulating equipment, 1 represents fluidised bed granulation and 2 is high shear granulation; and for the binder addition, 1 represents dry addition and 2 addition as a solution.

Various interconnections are possible in these data. The input formulation can be related to the granule properties as outputs. However, the granule properties can also be treated as inputs for examining the relationship to those of the finished tablets. The granule properties are intermediates in the formulation and, depending on the circumstances, may be treated either as inputs or as outputs. As can be seen in Figure 6.3, a variable can be defined as an Ingredient, a Property, or left as Not Used. Selecting the option Not Used is useful if it is necessary to exclude a particular variable from the training set without the necessity of removing it from the spreadsheet containing the input data. For example, by leaving mean granule size, flow value, bulk density and tap density as Not Used, a model connecting the input formulation directly to the properties of the finished tablet can be developed. In general, Not Used is very useful for examining the effect of leaving a particular variable out of the model. The option to specify variables as either ingredients or properties is also useful. For example, the granule properties can be treated as inputs in one model and as outputs in another model, again without the need to edit the original data set. Therefore, data input retains maximum flexibility.

6.3.4 *Training the Neural Network*

The process of developing a model linking inputs to outputs is referred to as training the neural net. CAD/Chem incorporates a number of neural network architectures and training algorithms organised into Basic and Advanced options. Hidden-layer architectures (with up to three hidden layers) are available with the option to specify the number of neurons in each of the hidden layers. Functional transformation of the input values is also allowed. For most formulation problems, the hidden layer network has been shown to be the most appropriate. It is generally accepted that about 85 per cent of all data sets will train adequately with a single hidden layer. All problems can be trained with more than one hidden layer but there is a risk of overtraining. In overtraining the network 'memorises' the data it is given and loses its predictive capability.

In addition to the hidden-layer architectures the Gaussian Functional Link Network can be used in CAD/Chem. This is a proprietary network of AI Ware Inc. and is a specific type of Radial Basis Function network as discussed in Chapter 5.

By default CAD/Chem develops a separate model for each output or property. This is the so-called Independent Outputs mode. An alternative, offered in the Advanced options, is Patterns of Cluster. In this case the data are first grouped according to a similarity criterion and a separate model is created for each sub-group or cluster. Patterns of Cluster may be the appropriate choice when measured properties are related, e.g. when one property is an average of two or three other property measurements.

6.3.5   *Architecture Selection*

Because it is designed to be used by formulators rather than neural network experts, CAD/Chem contains inbuilt rules for the selection of the neural networks and uses these to set up a default architecture which will minimise the risk of overtraining. This means that the novice user can safely select the default architecture and still expect to produce meaningful results. However, the expert user can still access the various network architectures and training algorithm options to explore the effect of making changes or to ensure that an optimum model is produced. Adding more neurons will increase the training time and may also result in overtraining so that the model loses its capacity for generalisation.

The criterion set within CAD/Chem for selection of a particular network architecture is:

$$\text{IF } [1.5n^2 + 3n + 1] < P \qquad \text{THEN } [\text{GFLN}]$$

where n is the number of inputs and P is the number of data records or experiments. For most formulation problems there are a significant number of inputs and a relatively small number of experiments so it is rare that the Gaussian Functional Link Network (GFLN) is the recommended choice.

For hidden-layer architectures, CAD/Chem also recommends the number of nodes to use in the hidden layer, based on the inequality:

No. of records > (No. of inputs) × (No. of hidden nodes + 1).

If this criterion cannot be met an architecture with one hidden layer, containing two neurons, is used as the default.

6.3.6   *Breaking Connections*

In general, each output will be connected to each input, possibly via the hidden layers. However, in some cases, there will be no relationship between changes in an input and an output and the user might wish to exclude any connection between the neurons in order to speed up the training process.

The CAD/Chem training workscreen contains a Connections button which provides access to a separate workscreen shown in Figure 6.4. This displays the Spearman rank coefficients connecting inputs to outputs both numerically and in a graphical form. If it is clear from other work that particular inputs are not correlated with outputs, the user might choose to disconnect these neurons either by selecting them individually or by setting a threshold value below which any connection will be ignored. This simplifies the overall connectivity of the network. However, it is generally useful to leave all the connections in place unless there is conclusive proof that there is no cause and effect relationship since, even when correlations are weak, there may be subtle interactions which affect the predicted properties.

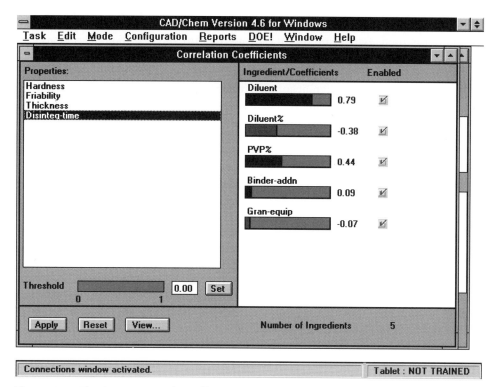

Figure 6.4 The Spearman rank coefficients give an indication of which properties and ingredients are correlated

6.3.7 *Selection of Training Algorithm*

Three different possibilities are incorporated within CAD/Chem for the training algorithm (discussed in Chapter 5). The default is Accelerated Back-propagation but simple back-propagation and conjugate gradient methods are also available. Simple back-propagation is generally slow but has been included in CAD/Chem so the user can compare with other neural network models. Conjugate gradient methods are slower than accelerated back-propagation but they are more likely not to stop in local minima and are guaranteed to converge given enough time and iterations. The advanced options within CAD/Chem let the user change the training algorithm and the relevant parameters, although sensible defaults are used so that the novice does not need to be concerned with these.

6.3.8 *Validation of Model*

A common complaint of using neural networks is that they are a 'black box'. Although a good model may be developed it is hard to assess how good it is. Since the prime requirement of the model is that it be able to predict 'unknown' data the usual approach is to keep back some of the data for validation. Within CAD/Chem these are referred to as 'test data' and there are facilities within the data spreadsheet both for manual and automatic selection of data records to be withheld for testing.

The rest of the data are used in the training of the neural network and the resulting model is then used to predict the properties for the test data. The degree of agreement between the measured and predicted properties, which is displayed on-screen during the training phase, gives a good measure of the predictive capability of the model. If there is a significant difference between the results for the training data and the test data the model is inadequate. The neural network architecture can be changed (usually simplified) to see whether better agreement can be found. This is the simplest method of model validation. Other courses of action for improving 'poor' models are discussed in Section 6.3.10.

Once the preferred architecture has been determined, it is advisable to train the network again, using all the data including that which was kept back for model validation. In this way the maximum information is extracted from the experimental data.

In newer releases of CAD/Chem, statistics relevant to the model can also be obtained by selecting a spreadsheet tab labelled Model Statistics. Standard ANOVA tables are given for every output model and the R^2 value (which describes how much of the variation in the data is accounted for in the model) is reported. Typically, an R^2 value of over 70 per cent indicates an adequate model and over 90 per cent denotes a good model. The f-ratio statistic, which indicates the extent to which the model fit exceeds the experimental error in the system, is also available. This is used in conjunction with the R^2 value to determine the goodness of the model and a value of at least 4 is usually required for the f-ratio. Because this information is readily accessible many of the concerns which more statistically-oriented formulators express about neural networks can be allayed.

6.3.9 The Tablet Formulation Example

In the case of the tablet formulation example, CAD/Chem defaults to a four-neuron single hidden layer network when 25 per cent of the data is held back for validation. Figure 6.5 shows the result of the training workscreen with each line corresponding to the model for a separate property. It can be seen that some of the models are denoted TRAINED(*), which indicates that a model is available but that it has not achieved the severe default threshold of 0.0001 which is set in CAD/Chem. This is in general not a problem and the user can set a less rigorous convergence criterion if desired.

6.3.10 Improving Poor Models

Occasionally it will be seen that the model does not train to the required accuracy and that predictive capability is poor. If the model has trained accurately but predicts badly then, as discussed above, reducing the complexity of the network (e.g. reducing the number of hidden-layer neurons) may solve the problem.

If the model is poorly trained it may be that there are questionable data. Examining the data for outliers and ensuring that the design space is reasonably well covered are useful first steps. The integrated analysis and graphics capabilities within CAD/Chem make this especially easy and questionable records can be removed or edited. If the data look sensible, it may be possible that an additional

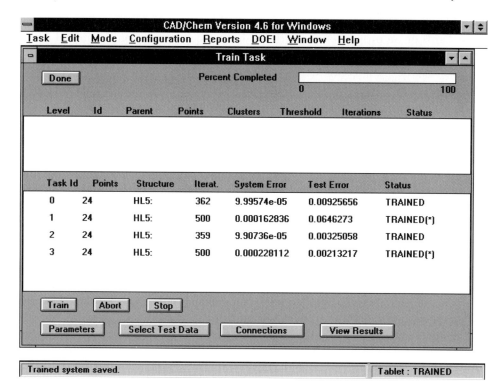

Figure 6.5 The training workscreen shows that all models exist, although some are marked TRAINED(*) indicating that they are not as accurate as requested

variable, which has not been measured, has a significant effect. This will lead to a significant amount of 'noise' in the data which may make the generation of an accurate model difficult or impossible. As with many modelling techniques, one of the most useful features of the modelling procedure is the ability to re-examine whether the data are sufficiently accurate and complete.

6.4 Using the Model

As mentioned above, CAD/Chem stores each trained model in a separate sub-directory in the working directory which was specified during installation. Therefore the model is accessible at any future time for the formulator to try out new ideas. Once the model is available any future access into CAD/Chem puts the user directly into the Consult mode, although it is possible for them to return to the other modes and load data or retrain the model as discussed in Section 6.2.

6.4.1 Retrieval of Previous Formulations

Frequently, an existing formulation is taken as the starting point for testing out further ideas. To make it easy to find a good starting point, CAD/Chem incorporates a Best Match feature which finds the closest match within the known data (using a Euclidean distance criterion) to the new formulation specified by the user.

Best Match can be used to retrieve the closest previous record by matching either on ingredients or on properties. Note that it has no dependence on the model which has been generated; it is simply a retrieval function working within known data.

6.4.2 *The Consult Mode*

As is clear from Figure 6.1, the model can be run 'forwards', making changes to the input conditions and seeing what effect this has on properties. A typical example is shown in Figure 6.6 which shows the Consult workscreen within CAD/Chem. Here the effect of changing the amount of PVP is under investigation, with the previous ingredients in the Found column and the new values, input by the user, in the Given column. The effect on the properties can be seen; previous properties are in the Given column, while the Found values show those which are predicted from the model. The calculations are virtually instantaneous even for the most complex formulations making it possible to test out a wide range of ideas very quickly.

Of course, a value needs to be provided for each of the ingredients for a sensible prediction to be made. If a particular ingredient is not used in the 'what if' experiment, then its value is set to zero. If a value is chosen which lies outside the range for any particular input, CAD/Chem will not perform the operation but will advise that 'System input is outside of data range'. As discussed earlier, extrapolation outside the known design space is possible but needs to be taken into account during the data loading phase so that the model is trained accordingly.

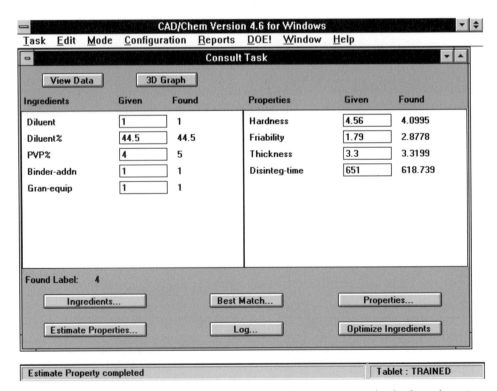

Figure 6.6 The Consult workscreen in CAD/Chem allows access to the facilities for using the model in 'what if' or optimisation modes

6.4.3 *The Optimisation Mode*

In general, optimising formulations is a complicated process because of the considerable number of interrelated variables which can be changed. Frequently, the desired properties are conflicting so that improving one will result in a degradation of another. Cost might also need to be taken into consideration. There will be constraints on the amount of materials that can be used and, possibly, on the process conditions. All of these taking place in a multidimensional design space make some sort of automation of the optimisation process essential.

The optimisation procedure in CAD/Chem involves setting up an objective function, which tries to satisfy the required properties (weighted by their relative importance) while allowing for any constraints on the ingredients including cost. The objective function has the form:

$$\frac{\sum_{i=1}^{P}(d_i(\text{property}_i).\,\text{weight}_i) + \text{weight}_{\text{cost}}.\,d_{\text{cost}}\left[\sum_{j=1}^{I}\text{ingredient}_j.\,\text{cost}_j\right]}{\sum \text{weight}}$$

(6.1)

where P is the number of properties, I is the number of ingredients and d is the desirability function for a property. All of the screens needed to set up the objective function are accessed using the Configuration button in the Optimisation screen of CAD/Chem shown in Figure 6.7. Four options can be set: costs, constraints on inputs, relative importance of properties, and desired values of properties.

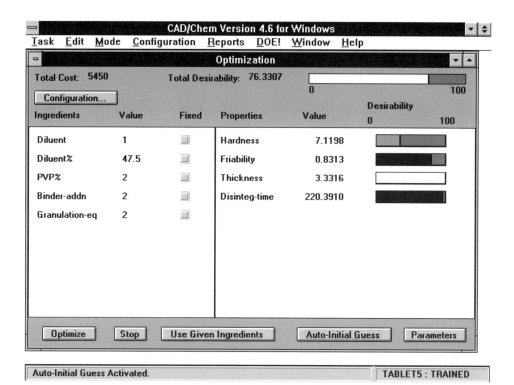

Figure 6.7 The Optimisation workscreen in CAD/Chem

Setting costs

The use of cost in the optimisation is optional and is switched on by the user as part of the optimisation parameter setup. By default, cost is not used in the optimisation and, in order to use it, the user must supply information on the cost of each ingredient. Cost can be used for process variables provided that it can be related to some meaningful unit, for example the running cost for a given period of time. If cost is used it can be weighted in importance just like any other property.

Setting property weights

In the case of formulations in which there are competing objectives – e.g. a strong tablet which also disintegrates rapidly – the specification of the relative importance of each property becomes crucial. These are the property 'weights' used in the equation and are on a scale of 1 (for least importance) to 10 (most important). Selecting a value of 0 is also possible but in this case it will have no effect on the objective function. The ability to weight each property differently on different occasions allows the user to 'tweak' formulations to meet different end-use applications most effectively.

Setting constraints

For some formulations there are constraints on the ingredients. These can be of various types. For example, a summation constraint would mean that the sum of a selected range of ingredients needs to add to a fixed value. In other cases there are inequality constraints, where the amount of one ingredient needs to be less/greater than another, or less/greater than a fixed value. There may also be constraints where a particular input must take an integral value. The tablet formulation example is a case in point. The granulation method can be either fluidised bed or high shear granulation and these have been denoted by the integers 1 and 2 respectively. A non-integral value – or indeed, any value other than 1 or 2 – has no meaning in this case. Constraints like these in which a variable needs to take discrete values, rather than continuous ones, can be set up using a modulus function.

One of the main constraints which should be used is that all the inputs lie within the region for which information has been gathered for the model development (neural network training) phase. Although it is possible to carry out an unconstrained optimisation, there are dangers in extrapolating outside the known design space especially if the model is significantly non-linear.

Setting desired property values

In Equation 6.1, each property is assigned a desirability value. When optimising a formulation to attain specific properties the user may wish a certain property to lie at the top end of the measured values, in the middle, or towards the minimum value, depending on the property. These can be set up quickly within CAD/Chem and setting desirabilities is the main function of the Desirability workscreen shown in Figure 6.8. The minimum and maximum values are filled in from the experimentally measured properties used in the training data set. The mid-point is simply an

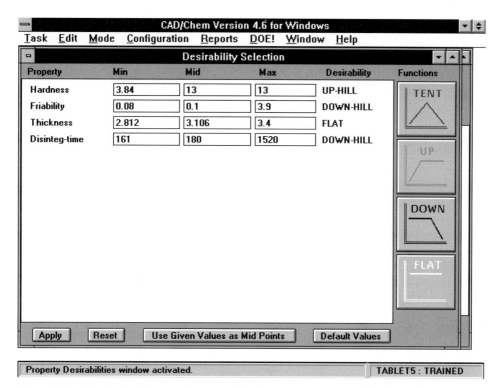

Figure 6.8 The Desirability workscreen, allowing customisation of the desired ranges of the optimised properties

average of the minimum and maximum points and can be edited by the user. This is useful in setting up the ranges which are desired for each property, for example, whether the property should lie towards the low end of the range, at the high end of the range, or at some intermediate value.

Icons are provided to help the user to set desired property values. They describe whether a property should lie between the minimum and the mid-point (Down-hill), between the mid-point and the maximum (Up-hill) or at the mid-point (Tent). If the user has no preferred value for the property and any value in the range is acceptable, the Flat icon can be chosen. Once the user has set up all the parameters to lie in the range of interest, the parameters can be applied by a single button press to accept the values.

Optimisation methods

Two optimisation methods are included within CAD/Chem. The default is Guided Evolutionary Simulated Annealing (GESA) which combines simulated annealing with genetic algorithms with the 'fitness' of each generation of solutions being a measure of how well it fits the user-defined objective function. GESA is an iterative procedure and the 'fittest' solutions get more 'children' in subsequent generations. GESA is very effective at finding the global minimum in the design space but may be time-consuming. As a result CAD/Chem searches only for 60 seconds before it stops. The user can set a different cut-off time if desired and can also start simulations for a further 60 seconds from the endpoint of the previous optimisation.

Because GESA is time-consuming, there is also an option to use the Flexible Tolerance Method (FTM) in which the design space is subdivided into polygons during the search. The FTM suffers from a disadvantage in that convergence may be to a local minimum, rather than the global optimum solution, hence GESA is usually preferred for complicated formulations.

The Optimisation and Consult workscreens are linked. Therefore, once the optimisation is complete, the values found are filled out on the Consult screen so that the user can return to carrying out 'what if' experiments or perform any of the other operations available from the screen.

6.5 Sensitivity Analysis

Having performed an optimisation and found a suggested formulation the user might wish to know how accurately the new ingredients need to be measured. This will depend on how susceptible the properties are to small changes in the ingredients and this can be determined by a sensitivity analysis.

The Consult workscreen has a button, View Data, which presents a spreadsheet containing the inputs together with the measured outputs, predicted outputs and percentage error. This spreadsheet contains a button for the Sensitivity. Users can choose the range for the variation in each input in terms of a percentage of its value. They can also choose whether the distribution around the input point is Gaussian, uniform, or fixed. Fixed might be an appropriate choice if, as is the case for binder addition in the tablet formulation example, non-integral values are not meaningful. The user is presented with a spreadsheet which shows the variation in the calculated properties as the ingredients are changed slightly; the information can be displayed graphically if required.

6.6 Graphical Display Reports

One of the useful features of any modern computer program is its ability to present information. CAD/Chem contains a number of graphical capabilities. Previously, it has been mentioned how data can be examined by looking at histograms and two- and three-dimensional plots in a variety of display styles. These can be useful in identifying questionable pieces of data or in ensuring that there is adequate coverage of the design space. Occasionally they may also reveal trends in the data.

These basic data display capabilities do not use the model in any way. However, the program also allows the user to examine 3D plots and contour plots which show the effect of different ingredients on a given property calculated using the neural network model. At present it is possible only to consider two ingredients and one property. One example, looking at the effect of both diluent percent and PVP percent on friability, is shown in Figure 6.9. Clearly these are simply 3D plots in a multidimensional design space and the model must use sensible values for the ingredients which are not displayed on the graph. The user has the option to use

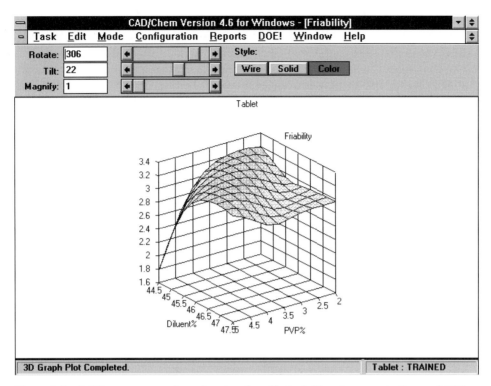

Figure 6.9 A 3D response surface showing the effect of diluent concentration and PVP concentration on tablet friability for the tablet formulation example. In this case, the diluent was lactose

the values from either the Given or the Found column of the Consult workscreen. The graphs can easily be transferred to the Windows clipboard and thereby into other applications such as word-processing packages or presentation graphics. Numerical reports of the points used in the display can also be obtained by selecting either the Table or Matrix options.

CAD/Chem also gives the option to present information in a variety of reports. From the pull-down Reports menu, the Optimisation report and the Correlation report (which summarises the Spearman rank coefficient used in setting up the model training) are generally regarded as the most useful. All of the reports are spreadsheet-enabled which means that they can be copied to the Windows clipboard and easily pasted into other applications.

CAD/Chem has a Notes facility which allows the user to type any relevant 'lab notes' to a file which is stored in the relevant subdirectory. This feature can be particularly useful for reminding the user of key features of the system and of the training and optimisation process when he or she returns to it at some future point.

Finally, CAD/Chem has a logging facility which allows the user to take a permanent note of a formulation of particular interest. If an optimisation, for example, suggests a new formulation, the user can log this via a button on the Consult workscreen. It will be date and time stamped and stored to the disk. The log is a spreadsheet with all the usual capabilities of CAD/Chem spreadsheets including graphical display and sensitivity analysis.

6.7 Conclusion

It can be seen that, although CAD/Chem is built on sophisticated technologies, its ease of use makes it readily accessible to formulators. Extensive on-line help and an optional 'Quick Tips' display provide assistance when needed. The integration of the graphical and analysis tools needed to understand and display the predictions from the model is an important feature of the program which further enhances its usefulness in new formulation design and optimisation.

References

1. KESAVAN, J.G. and PECK, G.E., 1995, Pharmaceutical formulation using neural networks, *Proc. 14th Pharm. Tech. Conf.*, **2**, 413–431.
2. COLBOURN, E.A. and ROWE, R.C., 1996, Modelling and optimization of a tablet formulation using neural networks and genetic algorithms, *Pharm. Tech. Eur.*, **8**, 46–55.

7

Knowledge Discovery and Data Mining

7.1 Introduction

It has been estimated that the amount of data in the world doubles every 20 months with the size and number of databases increasing at an even faster rate. Data is now stored at a rate that far outpaces the human ability to interpret and digest. Potentially valuable information and knowledge is hidden within these databases representing a missed opportunity since hidden knowledge could well provide a competitive advantage.

The solution to this problem lies in the rapidly emerging field of KDD (knowledge discovery in databases) and data mining. These two terms are not synonymous. The term KDD is often defined as:

> 'The non-trivial extraction of implicit, previously unknown and potentially useful information from data' (Frawley et al., 1991).

although to reflect the rapid growth in the field this definition has been recently revised to:

> 'The non-trivial process of identifying valid, novel, potentially useful and ultimately understandable patterns in data' (Fayyad et al., 1996a).

These definitions emphasise the overall process of discovering useful knowledge from data. Data mining, on the other hand, refers to the application of algorithms for extracting patterns from data. The term data mining has been commonly used by statisticians and data analysts but the term KDD has been mostly used by researchers in artificial intelligence and machine learning (Fayyad et al., 1996a).

7.2 Process and Technologies

An overview of the KDD process with data mining is shown in Figure 7.1. A rough breakdown of the relative amount of effort expended on the process is: problem identification, 10 per cent; obtaining/selecting data, 10 per cent; preprocessing data,

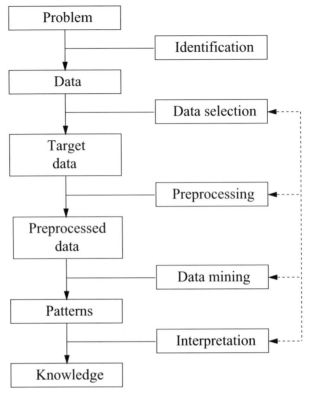

Figure 7.1   The knowledge discovery process as described by Fayyad *et al.* (1996a)

35 per cent; data mining, 30 per cent and interpretation of the results, 15 per cent (Roberts and Totton, 1996).

McClean and Scotney (1996) have viewed the data mining process in a somewhat different manner (Figure 7.2). They suggest a process in four steps:

- Data preprocessing where the data are cleansed and reformatted such that they are in the form appropriate to the mining algorithm. Typically data cleansing and missing value handling methods are used at this stage.
- Exploratory data analysis where the user has a preliminary look at the data to determine which attributes and technologies should be utilised. Typically visualisation methods are used at this stage.
- Data selection where the user focuses on certain attributes or groups of attributes. Typically clustering and classification methods are used at this stage.
- Knowledge discovery – the main objective in the process.

Whichever process is used, it is always interactive and iterative involving repeated application of specific methods or algorithms. The knowledge discovered can either be incorporated into an expert system in the form of rules or simply documented and reported to interested parties.

Data discovery/mining brings together the three disciplines of machine learning (including rule induction, neural networks, case-based reasoning and genetic algorithms), statistics and uncertainty methods (including linear regression, multivariate

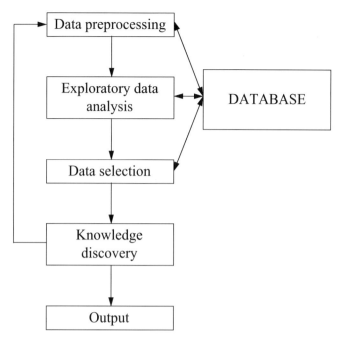

Figure 7.2   The data mining process as described by McClean and Scotney (1996)

analysis, principle component analysis, fuzzy logic and any other methods which are able to deal with imprecision and uncertainty) and database technology (including data cleansing, visualisation and other enabling technologies). Some techniques are particularly suited for specific types of problems but many may be less well suited for other application areas. Some techniques are useful for learning, others excel at explaining decisions: the field is limitless. For a full description of the technologies used in data discovery and data mining the reader is referred to *The Data Mining Report* by McClean and Scotney (1996).

7.3   Tools

Data mining tools can be either multi-paradigm embracing a number of different techniques/technologies or single paradigm embracing just one technique/technology. The former have been designed to provide methods which will be effective for a wide variety of application domains, the latter are generally associated with a particular potential application area, e.g. financial forecasting, predictive modelling.

Some data mining tools have been designed to be used directly with little formal training; others require considerable understanding of the technologies employed before they can be applied and are provided as part of a consultancy or implementation package. In all cases the tools are either interactive, requiring the input of knowledge from the domain expert, or automatic for non-technical users. Some offer the choice of interactive or automatic modes. A selection of data mining tools with suppliers is given in Table 7.1. All the tools are multi-paradigm embracing several techniques/technologies (Table 7.2). For a more detailed analysis the reader is referred to *The Data Mining Report* by McClean and Scotney (1996).

Table 7.1   Some representative examples of data mining tools and their suppliers

Tool	Supplier
Clementine	Integral Solutions Ltd
Data Engine	MIT GmbH
Data Logic	Reduct Systems Inc.
Data Mariner	Logica UK Ltd
IDIS	Information Discovery Inc.
Information Harvester	Information Harvesting Inc.
KATE	AcknoSoft
Knowledge Seeker	Angoss Software Int. Ltd
N-TRAIN/LOGIVOLVE	Scientific Consultant Services Inc.
RECALL	ISoft
SAS	SAS Software Ltd
SPSS	SPSS UK Ltd
XPERTRULE PROFILER	Attar Software Ltd

Table 7.2   A selection of data mining tools with their respective technologies (adapted from McClean and Scotney, 1996)

Tool	Technology					
	RI	CBR	NN	GA	FL	Stats
Clementine	X		X			
Data Engine	X		X		X	X
Data Logic	X			X		
IDIS	X	X			X	X
Information Harvester	X				X	X
KATE	X	X				X
Knowledge Seeker	X				X	X
N-TRAIN/LOGIVOLVE			X	X	X	X
RECALL	X	X				X
SAS			X			X
SPSS	X		X			X
XPERTRULE PROFILER	X					X

RI, rule induction; CBR, case-based reasoning; NN, neural network; GA, genetic algorithm; FL, fuzzy logic; Stats, statistics

Recently Brooks (1997) has suggested four criteria to be considered when choosing which tool(s) to use to solve a problem:

- Application domain – select the tool(s) appropriate to the problem to be addressed and the results to be obtained: no single tool is appropriate for all applications.
- Quantity of data – select the tool(s) that can process the amount of data that must be analysed.
- Resources – different tools require varying levels of resources, skills and time to be implemented.

- Price – product prices can range from hundreds of pounds to hundreds of thousands of pounds: generally the less expensive tools are more narrowly focused while the more expensive tools are more sophisticated and multi-paradigm.

Once several potential tools have been chosen, Brooks (1997) recommends that each be evaluated against real data. This is a necessary step because of the significant and unpredictable differences among different products and technologies.

7.4 Applications

Successful knowledge discovery and data mining applications are rarely made public, particularly if the discovered knowledge is used for competitive advantage. Successful applications have been developed in financial services, to analyse customer records (Callingham, 1997); retail stores to analyse turnover (Shearer, 1995); foreign exchange transactions (Shearer, 1995); astronomy to identify stars and galaxies (Fayyad *et al.*, 1996b); analytical chemistry to predict enantiomeric separation (Bryant *et al.*, 1995); transplant operations to identify factors affecting survival rates (Callingham, 1997); toxicology to predict skin corrosivity (Shearer, 1995) and to anticipate toxic hazards (Callingham, 1997); and many more (Totton *et al.*, 1995; Fayyad *et al.*, 1996a). A selection of applications where data mining tools have been explicitly stated is given in Table 7.3.

The following lessons have been learnt from these applications (Callingham, 1997):

- Data mining software is useless if it does not start with an understanding of real world problems.
- People with appropriate skills are required to deliver an answer; the technology is only as good as the people asking the questions.
- It is imperative that the correct data are collected.
- User friendly graphical user interfaces are a necessity and must integrate smoothly with the application environment.

Data mining, as such, has not been used in the domain of product formulation although the work done by Podczeck (1992) at the Martin-Luther University in

Table 7.3 A selection of applications of knowledge discovery/data mining where the software tool was explicitly stated

Field	Application	Tool
Analytical chemistry	Enantiomeric separation	Data Mariner
Financial services	Foreign exchange	Clementine
Health	Kidney transplants	Knowledge Seeker
Leisure	Market research	SPSS
Pharmaceutical	Tablet formulation	SPSS
Retail	Store turnover	Clementine
Toxicology	Skin corrosion	Clementine
Toxicology	Toxic hazards	Clementine

Table 7.4 Drugs and base mixture compositions analysed in the tablet formulation data mining application (Podczeck, 1992)

Drug	Dose (mg)
Acetylsalicylic acid (aspirin)	250
Caffeine	100
Codeine phosphate	30
Papaverine hydrochloride	100
Paracetamol (acetaminophen)	250
Phenacetin	250
Phenobarbitone	200
Phenylbutazone	200
Pholedrin sulphate	20
Propiprocaine hydrochloride	20
Propylphenazone	150
Quinidine hydrogen sulphate	125
Quinidine sulphate	100
Sodium salicylate	50
Theophylline	100

Base mixtures composition (% w/w)

	1	2	3
Microcrystalline cellulose (diluent)	90.60	89.05	15.10
Lactose (diluent)	–	–	69.97
Potato starch (disintegrant)	9.00	9.10	10.85
Colloidal silica (glidant)	–	1.60	3.48
Magnesium stearate (lubricant)	0.40	0.25	0.60

Granulation simplex composition	*(% w/w)*
Lactose (diluent)	30.0
Potato starch (disintegrant)	70.0

Granulated with a solution of 8% gelatin, 2% glycerol with magnesium stearate (lubricant) 0.3% added after addition of drug

Halle-Wittenberg, Germany using canonical analysis (a multivariate statistical method) to derive rules for a knowledge-based system for the formulation of tablets could be regarded as a form of data mining. In this application Podczeck (1992) analysed experimental data for 15 model drugs mixed with either three different basic mixtures or granulation simplex (Table 7.4) at five different concentrations (30, 40, 50, 60, 70% w/w) and then tabletted at three different compaction pressures (100, 200, 300 MPa). Weights of the formulations were adjusted to give the required dose of the drug(s) (Table 7.4) and the punch diameter varied between 5 and 13 mm depending on the weight of the tablet. Various granule and tablet properties were measured, as were a large number of physicochemical properties of the model drugs. The relationships found between drug, granule and tablet properties were then structured as a decision tree with rules allowing the prediction of a tablet formulation from a knowledge of the physicochemical properties of the drug. The system had 10 global rules with 524 specific rules. Examples of the global rules relating the physicochemical properties of the drug with the formulation are:

IF (bulk density of the drug is greater than 3.5 ml g^{-1})

THEN (use basic mixture 3 or granulation simplex)

and:

IF (no flowability)

THEN (basic mixture 1 is not suitable)

The system was tested with five new drugs: aminophylline (180 mg), ephedrine hydrochloride (50 mg), potassium chloride (250 mg), phenytoin (100 mg) and propranolol hydrochloride (25 mg) with the agreement between predicted and measured values being reasonable. Although in the paper the author did not give any details of the tool used it is believed that it was SPSS from SPSS UK Ltd (Table 7.1). Although relatively successful in demonstrating the use of such a software package, the system produced was never used, the author claiming the work to be only a contribution to fundamental research without any industrial use.

7.5 Conclusion

Knowledge discovery and data mining are still in the early stages of development despite the fact that many of the underpinning technologies are more established. There are no established criteria for deciding which methods to use in which circumstances, hence it is difficult to separate hype from reality. However there is no doubt that the potential benefits for the technology will ensure that it has a bright future. In this competitive age, data may well be a burden but the knowledge derived from it is likely to be an important asset well worth the resources spent acquiring it.

References

BROOKS, P.L., 1997, Keep your hands clean, *DBMS Magazine*, **2**(9), 35–42.

BRYANT, C.H., ADAM, A.E., CONROY, G.V., TAYLOR, D.R. and ROWE, R.C., 1995, Data Mariner, a commercially available data mining package and its application to a chemistry domain, *Data Mining*, **95**, 75–90, Uxbridge: Unicom Seminars Ltd.

CALLINGHAM, M., 1997, Data mining, *Business Computer World*, February, 80–86.

FAYYAD, U.M., PIATETSKY-SHAPIRO, G. and SMYTH, P., 1996a, From data mining to knowledge discovery: an overview, In FAYYAD, U.M., PIATETSKY-SHAPIRO, G., SMYTH, P. and UTHURUSAMY, R. (eds), *Advances in Knowledge Discovery and Data Mining*, pp. 1–34, Menlo Park, CA: AAAI Press.

FAYYAD, U.M., HAUSSLER, D. and STOLORZ, P., 1996b, KDD for science data analysis: issues and examples, *Proc. 2nd Int. Conf. Knowledge Discovery and Data Mining*, Menlo Park, CA: AAAI Press.

FRAWLEY, W.J., PIATETSKI-SHAPIRO, G. and MATHEUS, C.J., 1991, Knowledge discovery in databases: an overview, In PIATETSKI-SHAPIRO, G. and FRAWLEY, W.J. (eds), *Knowledge Discovery in Databases*, pp. 1–27, Cambridge, MA: AAAI/MIT Press.

McCLEAN, S. and SCOTNEY, B., 1996, *The Data Mining Report*, Uxbridge: Unicom Seminars Ltd.

PODCZECK, F., 1992, Knowledge based system for the development of tablets, *Proc. 11th Pharm. Tech. Conf.*, **I**, 240–264.

ROBERTS, H. and TOTTON, K., 1996, Data mining in BT, *Data Mining*, **96**, 224–232, Uxbridge: Unicom Seminars Ltd.

SHEARER, C., 1995, User-driven data mining applications, *Data Mining*, **95**, 70–74, Uxbridge: Unicom Seminars Ltd.

TOTTON, K., SHORTLAND, R. and SCARFE, R., 1995, Data mining applications in BT, *Data Mining*, **95**, 94–112, Uxbridge: Unicom Seminars Ltd.

8

Applications of Expert Systems – Non-Pharmaceutical

8.1 Introduction

There is now a wide variety of non-pharmaceutical products for which formulation expert systems have been applied (Table 8.1). This does not assume that all these products are now formulated using fully developed and integrated systems. In many cases, only prototype systems are described in the literature as many companies are reticent to publish openly on their applications. To the author's knowledge no comprehensive survey has ever been carried out on laboratories known to be working in this area, but a cursory inspection of current literature does reveal that it would include many important companies as well as some academic and government laboratories. In this chapter published applications from a variety of fields are reviewed.

8.2 Agrochemicals

An essential part of the development of a new agrochemical (e.g. pesticide, herbicide, fungicide, etc.) is the establishment of a formulation which is:

- effective in that the active ingredient has the maximum desired biological effect with minimum adverse side effects;
- convenient for the customer use;
- safe for the user and the environment;
- stable both chemically and physically under the conditions of use;
- easily manufactured;
- inexpensive or has an acceptable cost;
- acceptable to regulatory bodies.

Table 8.1 Examples of non-pharmaceutical products to which formulation expert systems have been applied

Field	Product	Development tool	Company
Agrochemicals	Emulsifiable concentrates	LISP Knowledge Craft PFES	Rohm and Haas Schering Agrochemicals (now AgrEvo)
Coatings	Paints Varnishes Resins	PROLOG PFES	BASF Exxon Chemicals ICI (UK)
Foods	Relishes Soft drinks Szechwan cooking	PFES CBR	
Personal care	Suncare products	PFES	Boots Company (UK)
Textiles	Wool dyeing Textile finishing		Sandoz (now Clariant)
Specialties	Adhesives Aluminium alloys Cleaning agents Dyestuffs Inks Lubricating oils Plastics Vinyl coatings Vinyl pipes	PROLOG Insight 2+ Knowledge Craft Knowledge Pro PFES	ALCOA Schering Industrial Chemicals Shell Research (UK) US Army Zeneca Specialties

For pharmaceutical products and companies see Chapter 9

There are three basic formulation types: dry powder systems, which include dusts, wettable powders and water-dispersible granules; water based systems which include emulsion concentrates, soluble liquid concentrates and suspension concentrates; and liquid systems based on polar organic solvents which include emulsifiable concentrates.

- **Dusts** – consist of the active ingredient co-milled with carriers. They are easy and cheap to produce, convenient to use but have a high potential risk of user contamination. Their physical stability can be affected by damp conditions.

- **Wettable powders** – consist of the active ingredient mixed with a carrier, wetting agent and dispersant. They are cheap to produce, easy to handle with few stability problems. When properly diluted they form a uniform suspension of fine particles.

- **Water-dispersible granules** – consist of the active ingredient mixed with a carrier, wetting agent and dispersant. They are easy and safe to handle, easy and cheap to package with few stability problems. They produce less dust than wettable powders.

- **Emulsion concentrates** – consist of the active ingredient, an emulsifier, an antifreeze, a stabiliser and an organic solvent presented as an oil-in-water emulsion. They are very effective, contain very little solvent, are cheap to produce and can be very stable.

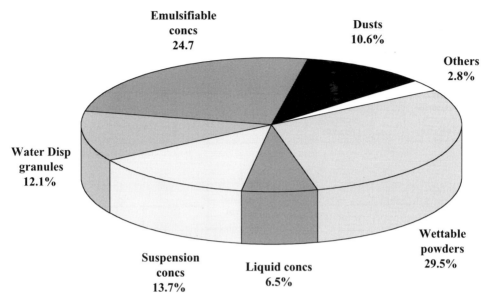

Figure 8.1 Distribution (by volume) of pesticide sales of different formulation types for agrochemicals in the European Union for 1989 (Smith, 1995)

- **Soluble (liquid) concentrates** – contain the active ingredient with a wetting agent and a surfactant dissolved in water. They are cheap and easy to produce but cannot contain high concentrations of active ingredient due to problems with crystallisation. They are also susceptible to freezing.

- **Suspension concentrates** – often called flowables, these systems are relatively complex formulations consisting of the active ingredient, a diluent, a wetting agent, a dispersant, a thickener, an anti-foaming agent and an antifreeze dispersed in water. They can contain very high concentrations of active ingredient, are easy to use but can settle out on storage.

- **Emulsifiable concentrates** – solvent based formulations which consist of the active ingredient and emulsifier(s) designed to form a stable emulsion when diluted with water. Their high solvent content increases their flammability and toxicity towards users. However, they are easy to produce and versatile.

Until the 1940s virtually all agrochemicals were applied as dusts. Wettable powders and emulsifiable concentrates began to appear in the 1950s with suspension concentrates and water-dispersible granules being introduced in the 1970s. Figure 8.1 shows the frequency distribution of formulation types for pesticides in the European Union in 1989 (Smith, 1995). It is not surprising that the first recorded reference to an expert system for the formulation of agrochemicals included information on five of these formulation types (dusts were excluded) although only a system for emulsifiable concentrates was developed. The overall structure of that system designed by personnel at Rohm and Haas is shown in Figure 8.2 (Hohne and Houghton, 1986).

The system was written in LISP to follow the natural structure of the formulation problem. For each problem area, data were acquired by consulting with the user or, in some cases, by accessing external programs. The system then used forward chaining to provide a series of hypotheses which were then sorted and

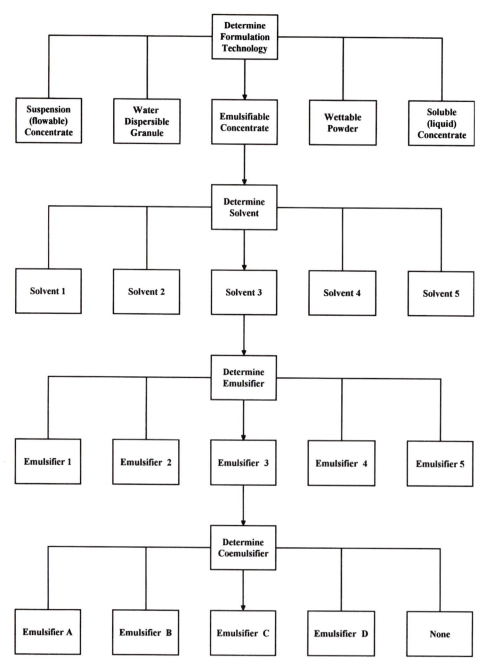

Figure 8.2 Structure of the agrochemical formulation problem as used by Hohne and Houghton (1986)

ranked. Backward chaining and a depth-first search routine was used to define what additional data are required before a definitive choice was made (Figure 8.3). At all times the user could override the system's choice if desired. The system also used production rules with confidence factors in the THEN clause. An example of the type of rule used is as follows:

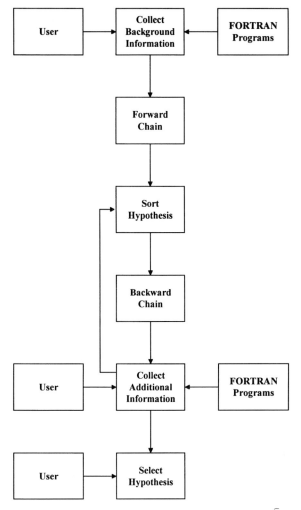

Figure 8.3 Strategy as used by Hohne and Houghton (1986) for agrochemical formulation

IF (concentration of active ingredient > 40%)

THEN (cannot formulate an emulsifiable concentrate) (0.5)

AND (cannot formulate a soluble concentrate) (0.5)

AND (cannot formulate a suspension concentrate) (0.5)

BECAUSE (concentration of active ingredient too high for these formulations)

i.e. there is a 50 per cent probability that at concentrations of active ingredient above 40 per cent these types cannot be formulated successfully.

The system was interfaced to two FORTRAN programs, one a molecular modelling program whereby the formulator could enter the chemical structure of the active ingredient which was then broken down into its functional groups, the second which calculated, using group contribution theory, the solubility of the active ingredient in a group of solvents. These programs were already in use by the synthetic chemists and their incorporation within the formulation expert system was

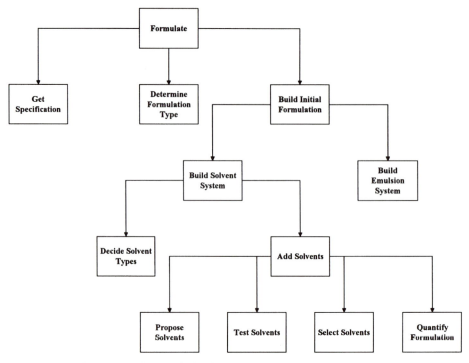

Figure 8.4 Task structure for emulsifiable concentrates

seen as a distinct advantage. At the time of publication, the knowledge base only contained rules to formulate an emulsifiable concentrate although further enhancements were discussed (Hohne and Houghton, 1986).

It is interesting to note that this same application was also investigated by personnel at Schering Agrochemicals Ltd UK (now AgrEvo) and Logica UK Ltd under the UK Alvey Programme (1987). The prototype system had two functions: to choose the formulation type; and to choose and quantify the ingredients for emulsifiable concentrates, although a limited amount of work was also done on wettable powder formulations in order to verify that a second type of formulation would fit into the structure of the prototype. The hierarchy of formulation tasks relevant to the development of emulsifiable concentrates is shown in Figure 8.4.

Knowledge acquisition was carried out using interviews with one domain expert and two knowledge engineers. Three basic types of interviews were used:

- General interviews where the expert was allowed to describe the domain.
- Focused interviews where the knowledge engineers posed detailed questions on the domain.
- Case histories where the expert presented case studies to illustrate a specific aspect of the domain.

Each interview was of approximately 90 minutes duration and recorded on audio tape. The tapes were then transcribed into notes – a process that took on average 4.5 hours per tape – at a rate of one tape per day. In constructing the prototype, knowledge elicitation, analysis and refinements required six man-months of the expert's effort, amounting to 30 per cent of the total time expended.

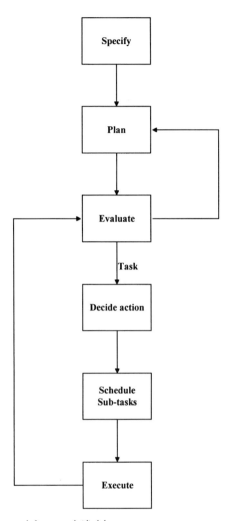

Figure 8.5 Strategy as used for emulsifiable concentrates

The system was implemented using Knowledge Craft from the Carnegie Group Inc. The design of the system was divided into three levels, each concerned with different aspects of the knowledge used by the domain expert. The top level, called the strategy level, dealt with the control, monitoring and problem solving tasks; the middle, called the design level, dealt with the building of the formulation; and the bottom level, called the physical level, dealt with the factual knowledge.

The structure of the strategy level is shown diagrammatically in Figure 8.5. The user's specification of the problem resulted in the generation of a series of plan steps each of which was processed in turn. The formulation was evaluated with respect to the targets relevant to the plan step and an action proposed which was subsequently broken down into sub-tasks. These were then executed and the formulation re-evaluated. If all targets were met, the next step was progressed, otherwise another action was proposed and the process continued.

The design level consisted of two sub-levels, one comprising operators which took an action from the strategy level and derived a set of steps to achieve it, the

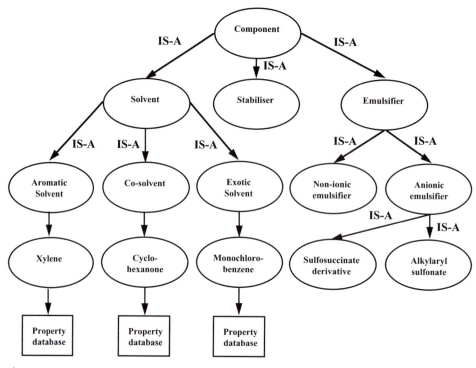

Figure 8.6 Semantic network for a selection of the components database used for emulsifiable concentrates

second comprising operators which dealt with construction of the formulation i.e. the choice of the most suitable ingredient or running a particular test.

The physical level comprised the facts, concepts and relationships relevant to the domain i.e. all the factual domain knowledge as distinct from the problem-solving knowledge. Figure 8.6 illustrates a section of the components database in the system in the form of a semantic network. The component hierarchy consisted of a set of frames representing either an individual component or a class or a system of components. Each component in the hierarchy contained slots representing the attributes or properties of that component. For solvents these properties included flash point, boiling point, specific gravity, EPA code and status and cost.

A feature of the agrochemical prototype was the inclusion of a mechanism for recording the progress of the formulation. This was necessary, first to allow backtracking when lines of development prove fruitless, second to provide an explanation of how the formulation was reached, and third to allow variations to be developed without repeating all the original work. The mechanism used to do this was present in the Knowledge Craft tool-box.

The prototype, although sufficiently well developed for demonstration purposes, fell short of requirements for an operational system. However, it did demonstrate that agrochemical formulation knowledge and expertise could be embodied in an expert system. The lessons learnt led to the ultimate development of the PFES kernel (Chapter 3) and an agrochemical formulation expert system based on this software. For a detailed description of the agrochemical application the reader is referred to Volume 2 of the Alvey Project Report (1987).

8.3   Aluminium Alloys

High purity aluminium is soft and lacks strength but its alloys, containing small amounts of other elements (e.g. copper, magnesium, iron, silicon, chromium, lead, lithium, etc.), are much stronger and formable by many metal-working processes. They can be joined, cast, machined and accept a wide variety of finishes. The properties of aluminium alloys depend on their microstructure which is controlled both by the chemical composition and by processing. In addition to features such as voids, inclusions and dislocations present in all metallic products, aluminium alloys are characterised by three types of intermetallic particles referred to as constituent particles (formed during solidification), dispersoids (formed during thermal treatment of an ingot by precipitation of a solid solution) and precipitates (formed during heat treatment of the final mill product by precipitation from a supersaturated solid solution). The nature of the constituent, dispersoid and precipitated particles depends strongly on the phase diagram of the particular alloy (Staley and Haupin, 1992).

The alloy design or formulation problem begins with the specification required for the physical properties of the product. In order to achieve this the designer or formulator selects a known material that has properties similar to the design target. These are then altered by making changes to the composition and processing methods in steps. Often these do not result in the desired end properties and, in these cases, the designer constructs a model of the microstructure that will produce the required properties (Gupta and Ghosh, 1988). Alloy design in an industrial ·setting involves a team of expert metallurgists each of whom is a specialist in a different technical area. It is not surprising, therefore, that this domain was one of the first to be targeted for a product formulation expert system.

The expert system developed by Rychener *et al.* (1985) known as ALADIN (ALuminium Alloy Design INventor) is one of the few complete and one of the most successful systems known. Developed for ALCOA (Aluminium Corporation of America) it served two major functions: a decision support system in suggesting the composition, processing methods or microstructural features necessary to meet a suggested specification; and as a design assistant in producing an evaluation of a given design or formulation.

Implemented using Knowledge Craft from the Carnegie Group Inc., ALADIN used multispatial reasoning architecture based on five spaces (Figure 8.7):

- Property space containing knowledge of alloy properties.
- Structure space containing knowledge of alloy microstructures.
- Composition space containing knowledge of different alloying elements (e.g. magnesium, copper, silicon, etc.).
- Process space containing knowledge of all thermo-mechanical alloy manufacturing processes.
- Metaspace containing knowledge about design process and control strategies.

Each space had its own search space, hypotheses and abstraction levels. The metaspace was of strategic importance in that planning and search took place in this space after generating the decision trees of various alternatives. Activity was generated at three levels or planes: a meta or strategic plane which planned for the design process itself establishing sequencing, priorities, etc.; a structure planning plane which formulated targets of the alloy microstructure in order to realise the

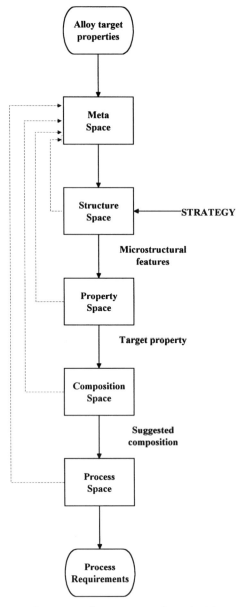

Figure 8.7 Multispacial architecture of ALADIN as described by Rychener *et al.* (1985)

desired macro-properties; and an implementation plane which encompassed the composition and processing spaces.

The alloy design problem typically started in the structure space with decisions on the microstructural features that implied desired properties. These decisions were then implemented in the composition and process space. A problem with any multistage system like ALADIN is that a decision optimal at one stage may be infeasible at a subsequent stage. This was dealt with in the system architecture using search processes that employed a least commitment principle i.e. values within hypotheses were expressed as ranges that were kept as broad as possible.

112

ALADIN used three forms of knowledge representation:

- Declarative knowledge consisting of a database of physical properties, compositions and processing methods, structured using frames and inheritance. For the description of microstructure which, in practice, generally involved the visual inspection of micrographs, a symbolic representation involving the enumeration of types and size of particles and dislocations was developed. This allowed microstructural facts to be expressed even if quantitative data were unavailable.

- Production rules which were used throughout the system for control of search, association of causes, processing of user commands and decisions about when to call on other knowledge spaces. An example of a simple production rule from ALADIN was:

  IF (magnesium is added)

  THEN (strength will increase)

- Algorithms which were used for statistical, chemical and thermomechanical calculations. These numeric computations were coupled with symbolic reasoning based on heuristic knowledge that estimated the relative advantage and accuracy of the choices made.

ALADIN had a model of alloy design strategy that was encoded in production rules and associated with the metaspace. The system began in the metaspace and frequently returned there for new direction. When the metaspace was activated, strategic rules identified activities that were reasonable and created top level goals in memory. These goals were expanded by creating sub-goals. These goal trees constituted a plan, control of which then returned to the structure, property, composition or process spaces which processed the goals. Iteration between the meta and domain spaces continued until the problem was solved.

Rychener *et al.* (1985) described the system as a 'mature advanced prototype' with a typical design run taking approximately an hour. At that time plans were well advanced to refine and extend the knowledge base away from the original focus on three additives, two microstructural aspects and five design properties. The project was, and still is, regarded as a major success in the application of formulation expert systems. For a detailed description of ALADIN the reader is referred to Rychener *et al.* (1985) and the references therein.

8.4 Inks

An ink can be defined as a complex formulation of colouring matter dispersed in a vehicle or carrier, which forms a fluid or paste which can be printed on a substrate and dried (Bassemir *et al.*, 1995). The colorants are generally pigments, toners, dyes or combinations of these selected to provide the desired colour contrast. The vehicle is generally a varnish or polymeric resin (e.g. acrylics, alkyds, cellulosics, vinyls) dispersed or dissolved in an oil (e.g. vegetable or mineral) and/or a solvent (e.g. alcohols, hydrocarbons, esters, ketones or water) designed to act as a carrier for the colorant during the printing operation and, in most cases, to serve to bind the colorant to the substrate. Other ingredients added to the formulation include driers, waxes, lubricants, surfactants, thickeners, gellants, defoamers, antioxidants and preservatives.

Inks vary considerably in composition, physical appearance, method of application and drying mechanism. They may be pastes (e.g. lithographic inks) or liquids (e.g. flexographic and rotogravure inks) but all require careful formulation to achieve their optimum end use properties of drying rate, tackiness, viscosity, colour and gloss. The world ink industry in 1992 had total sales in excess of $10.5 billion of which the USA had sales of $2.92 billion. More than 60 per cent of these sales were made by the top ten ink producers which accounted for only 4 per cent of the total number of ink companies in the USA (Bassemir *et al.*, 1995).

It is not surprising that in such a diverse and fragmented field the use of formulation expert systems has been critically evaluated. In 1987, Stone (1987) of BASF first introduced the concept by discussing the formulation of a general purpose let-down varnish for heat-set inks. Three parts of the problem were evaluated: the selection of a gellant; the selection of a solvent; and the selection of a resin. Code written in TURBO PROLOG for all three parts was given in the text. A flow diagram for the selection of a resin is shown in Figure 8.8. First the expert system attempted to select from the database a resin having properties close to that required. If none were available, a binary mixture was chosen such that the properties of one resin compensated for the deficiencies of the other. Calculations were used to predict the properties of the mixture. Failure to meet any of the required properties forced the system to backtrack and look for other solutions. Even if the mixture was satisfactory, the system looked for alternatives. Although an oversimplification of the problem, all three systems served to illustrate the applicability of expert systems to ink formulation.

In 1990, personnel at Exxon, a supplier of raw materials to the ink industry, produced an expert system called INFORM, a generalised ink formulation assistant based on in-house investigations on how varnishes for offset inks were formulated (Frisch *et al.*, 1990). Implemented using Knowledge Pro from Knowledge Garden Inc. together with PROLOG for the search routines, INFORM used a collection of rules to represent the formulation knowledge of the expert. These rules constituted the database which related components of the formulation (e.g. resins and solvents/ solvent composition) to the properties of the ink (e.g. viscosity, tack, tack rise, gloss, etc.). Using previously published measurements and input from formulators, rules which defined how each component affected each property of interest in qualitative terms were generated. The system as described contained ten components, nine properties and four qualitative descriptors of effect (Figure 8.9).

The formulator applied these rules to a problem by specifying a primary property together with several secondary properties that needed to be modified (increased, decreased or maintained) to achieve a desired endpoint. INFORM then produced recommendations using a 'generate and test' method i.e. it created a branch on a search tree and then checked whether there had been a positive impact on the primary property. If the result was positive, it then examined the impact on the secondary properties. If the cumulative net impact was good then the new formulation was regarded as being acceptable. Using a depth-first search mechanism INFORM ultimately produced a list of possible solutions which were then differentiated by a scoring routine. This was based on numerical scores defining the relative changes in a property resulting from a change in the component e.g. a significant change

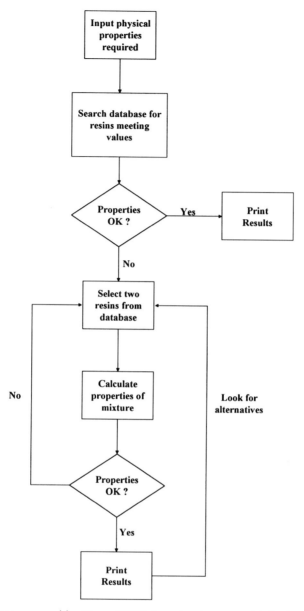

Figure 8.8   Strategy as used by Stone (1987) for a let-down varnish for heat-set inks

was given two points, a slight change one point and unknown/no change zero points. If the direction of the change was desirable the score was positive, if undesirable the score was negative. Cumulative scores for each recommendation were then generated. Choice of a threshold value then resulted in a list of the best formulation options to solve the problem in hand.

The system was regarded by its developers as being successful in that it fully achieved three goals set for it: a receptacle for in-house expertise; a training tool to improve effectiveness; and an interactive tool to solve customers' problems (Frisch *et al.*, 1990).

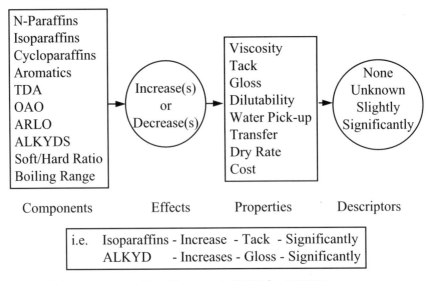

Figure 8.9 Rule structure used by Frisch *et al.* (1990) for INFORM

8.5 Lubricating Oils

A typical lubricating oil consists of a base oil to which can be added up to ten chemical additives chosen from a large database. The common types of additives include oxidation inhibitors, corrosion inhibitors, antiwear agents, friction modifiers, detergents, dispersants, viscosity improvers, pour-point depressants and foam inhibitors (Booser, 1995). Some additives combine several functions, e.g. zinc dialkyl dithiophosphate (ZDTP) is both an oxidation inhibitor and an antiwear agent, and interaction between additives (e.g. ZDTP and some detergents) can lead to both beneficial and deleterious effects. Additives are present in quantities ranging from a few parts per million to several percent. They can also be expensive relative to the cost of the base oil and since lubricating oils are a large volume product any reduction in the amount and cost of the additives used could result in large savings.

Central to lubricating oil formulation is the use of engine tests to evaluate performance. This is because the physical and chemical processes that take place within a modern engine and which influence the performance of the formulation are poorly understood. In addition no single engine test can reproduce all of the potential operating conditions. Hence engine testing is both time consuming and expensive and there is a strong incentive to minimise its unnecessary use.

Formulating lubricating oils is thus an expensive, time consuming process involving the highest levels of decision making. Hence its choice as the second application in the UK Alvey Programme involving Shell Research Ltd UK and Logica UK Ltd (1985–1987).

The task structure of the prototype developed for lubricating oil formulation is shown in Figure 8.10. This structure has two interesting features. First, it was not fixed but varied from problem to problem both in the order in which the tasks were performed and also the tasks were not entirely independent because of the possible interactions between components. In addition the system was structured to avoid making premature decisions until the antiwear additives had been considered.

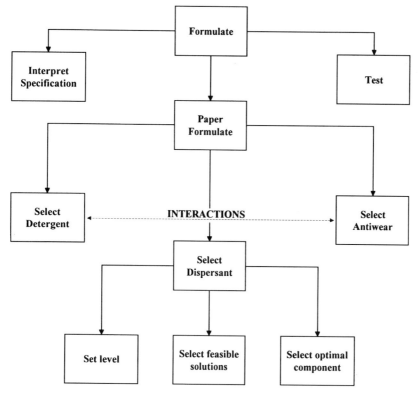

Figure 8.10 Task structure for lubricating oil formulations

Since there are no textbooks on formulating lubricating oils considerable time and effort was expended on the acquisition of formulation knowledge. Approximately 50 interviews averaging about one hour took place over a period of 18 months. Early interviews involving one or two domain experts and three or four knowledge engineers were loosely structured. However later interviews on a one-to-one basis were planned to elicit both the declarative and procedural knowledge. Interviews were recorded and transcribed for future reference.

Since it was considered that lubricating oil formulation in its entirety was too broad a problem to be tackled in one go, rapid prototyping of various subsets was tried. This was implemented in Knowledge Craft from the Carnegie Group Inc. with LISP for encoding rules. The third prototype designed to produce a paper formulation for a lubricating oil to meet typical standard specifications with an extension to incorporate reformulation was the first to be shown in detail to the formulators.

Although this system fulfilled its role as a test bed for research ideas and demonstrated the feasibility of a number of key ideas especially around knowledge elicitation and representation, it was of very limited value in reproducing the activities of a formulator in this field. For a detailed evaluation of the project the reader is referred to Volume 2 of the Alvey Project Report (1987).

As a consequence of the project, personnel at Shell Research Ltd UK have re-implemented some of the key concepts specifically on explicating the reasoning process and making it accessible and modifiable to the formulators (Lunn *et al.*,

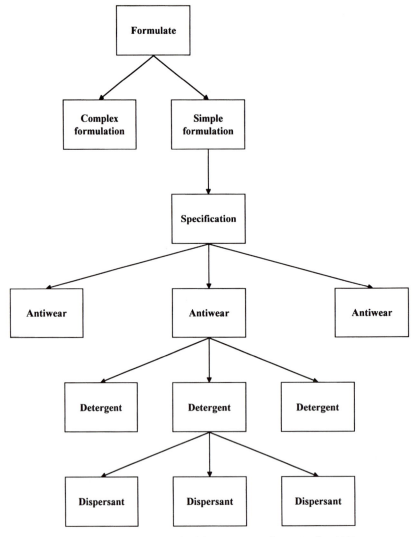

Figure 8.11 Formulation tree as described by Lunn *et al.* (1991) for ALF

1991). A new system, ALF (Artificial Lubricant Formulator), has been implemented in QUINTUS PROLOG with an interfacing tool called Prowindows.

The system produced a formulation tree with various tasks (Figure 8.11). Attached to each node was a pop-up menu which allowed the formulator to enact a task. For example, the 'formulate' node offered two options, 'simple formulate' or 'complex formulate'; the 'simple formulate' mode offered the tasks 'specify' (a constraint on the wear value), 'zinc' (an antiwear additive) and 'detergent' and 'dispersant'. The system also included a causal network whereby the formulator could instantly view the interaction between the components and effects and their hierarchy. Links were tagged with integers in the range −5 to +5 to infer the degree of causation. A causal network editor has also been constituted to provide an adequate means to present and edit the knowledge.

The system has been used to complement the decision making of a formulator but is not seen as a replacement. It is regarded as a useful tool (Lunn *et al.*, 1991).

8.6 Propellants

Propellants are mixtures of chemical compounds that produce large volumes of high temperature gas at controlled, predetermined rates with the principle application of launching projectiles from guns, rockets and missile systems. Typical components include an oxidiser of the nitramine, nitro or nitrate ester type; a binder, often a polymeric ester; and various other additives such as stabilisers, flash suppressants, inhibitors, lubricants, processing aids, etc. Factors influencing the selection of components include energy delivery, burn rate, temperature dependence and decomposition temperature, stability on storage, reliability, manufacturability and cost (Lindner, 1993). Formulation in this domain is very much driven by intuition and is not documented. In addition the recent development of new materials has resulted in a large increase in the number of possible combinations of ingredients.

Using the Insight 2+ shell from Level Five Research, Shaw and Fifer (1988) from the US Army Ballistic Research Laboratories have developed an expert system for the formulation of nitramine propellants. Insight 2+ was chosen since it was easy to interface with the current databases of propellant ingredients and their properties. This was seen as critical to the development of the system since some of the computation involved estimating propellant properties which could not be carried out from within the rules. Knowledge was expressed as production rules with backward chaining.

The expert system was developed in separate modules. Figure 8.12 is a schematic representation of the operation and interaction of the various modules. The pre-screening module queried the user for all necessary information including requirements for the formulation (energy, burn rate, cost, etc.) and specific ingredient preferences if any. This was a highly interactive process with access to explanations and lines of reasoning. The user specified requirements/preferences and these were then used by rules to search the individual databases (oxidisers, binders, plasticisers) in series for components which met the desired criteria. The positives were then saved in their respective reduced databases or datafiles. A formulation generator was then used to generate ingredient combinations and reject others. Acceptable combinations were then written to a textfile. Concentrations of the various ingredients were set semi-quantitatively in terms of high, medium and low levels generating nine formulations in total. Properties for all these formulations were extracted using both production rules (for burn rate, cost, etc.) and external programs (for energy properties) before the formulations plus properties were written to a database for interrogation by the user.

Despite the use of rules to narrow down the number of ingredients and ingredient combinations the number of formulations in the formulation database could be quite large. Using the interrogation module, the formulator could ask for reports on, for instance, the ten cheapest formulations or the ten highest energy formulations.

At the time of writing, the authors reported that all modules were functional and interactive and that further work was being undertaken to expand the system. It is interesting to note that rule induction using the 1st Class shell was being applied to the problem (Shaw and Fifer, 1988).

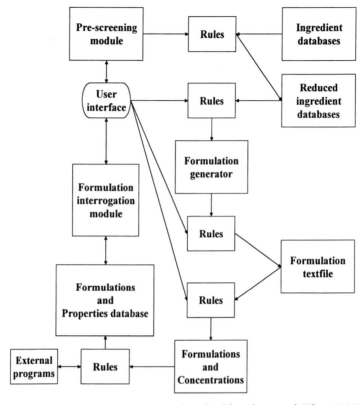

Figure 8.12 Structure of the expert system described by Shaw and Fifer (1988) for propellant formulation

8.7 Suncare Products

Sun protection is now a major issue throughout the world. Investigations of the impact of ultraviolet light over the wavelength ranges from 285–320 nm (UVB) and between 330 nm and visible light (UVA) have demonstrated its potential to burn skin resulting, not only in tanning and sunburn but also in the production of more damaging long term effects such as melanoma. High sun protection factor (SPF) values and the provision of broad spectrum protection are now important factors in the formulation of suncare products. To achieve the higher SPF values demanded normally requires a cocktail of organic and inorganic (micronised oxides) absorbers and care must be taken that they stay within the restrictions imposed by relevant legislative bodies. In addition small changes in the formulation can dramatically affect SPF values.

Although SPF values undoubtedly have a bearing on the purchase decision of the customer, other factors such as appearance, skin feel, fragrance (if any), application properties and price are also important and must be considered by the formulator. A product that spreads easily on the skin may not leave sufficient film thickness to achieve its expected performance. Ideally a formulation should spread readily under shear but instantly regain viscosity after application, forming an even film.

Formulation of suncare products is thus a highly skilled occupation requiring three to four years of experience to attain a reasonable level of experience. Consequently in 1991 personnel from the Boots Company Ltd UK and Logica UK Ltd developed an expert system to assist formulators in this domain. Implemented using PFES from Logica (Chapter 3) the system, called SOLTAN, used knowledge captured from senior formulators. Ingredients, processes and relationships of the formulation were represented in a way that reflected their groupings and associations in the real world and existing information sources, such as databases, were presented in a frame-based semantic network which could be manipulated by the problem solving knowledge of the domain. Tasks were structured in a hierarchy which was built up dynamically depending on the specification in hand as the problem solving process proceeded. Knowledge about the formulation was distributed throughout the task hierarchy with strategic knowledge represented towards the top of the hierarchy and tactical knowledge towards the bottom.

The system was originally developed to formulate sun oils (solutions of ultraviolet absorbers in emollients) but was rapidly extended, with the incorporation of basic emulsion technology, to cover oil-in-water lotions. Subsequently the system was further expanded to incorporate water-in-oil, oil-in-water and water-in-silicone creams and lotions. It can now be used to formulate all types of skincare products, not just suncare products (Wood, 1991). The system won second prize in the DTI Manufacturing Intelligence Awards in 1991.

8.8 Textile Finishing

Finishing of textiles includes, in its broadest sense, any process used to improve a knitted, woven, or bonded textile fabric for apparel or other home or industrial use (Vail, 1983). Finishing processes vary widely because of the great differences in the chemical and physical properties of the fibres available. In 1992, Frie and Poppenwimmer estimated that there were 140 manufacturers of chemicals in Europe offering 7000–8000 different products for the finishing of textiles. Their own company, Sandoz (now Clariant), offered approximately 330 different chemicals for textile refinement and approximately 100 for finishing (Frie and Poppenwimmer, 1992). It is on this basis that the authors developed an expert system for textile finishing called TEXPERTO (Frie and Poppenwimmer, 1992).

The system, outlined in Figure 8.13, recommended customer specific formulations based on rules derived from experts in textile finishing with Sandoz, Switzerland. TEXPERTO used, as its starting point, a detailed description of the textile in terms of its group (e.g. clothing, textiles for the house and home, and others), subdivided into individual article groups (e.g. outerwear, linen, lining/padding, scarves, sport/leisure, etc.) as well as its important characteristics (e.g. fibre, structure, white component, washing instructions and aftercare requirements). The system then requested the effects to be achieved by the finishing process (e.g. texture, stain protection, sewability, wash and wear, white component and white nuance) as well as recommending others that could be considered based on the textile description.

Since it is well known that the process also plays an important role in defining the final formulation, TEXPERTO also recommended typical processing steps which could either be accepted by the user or changed to suit specific requirements. Furthermore the user could set restrictions on the selection of ingredients

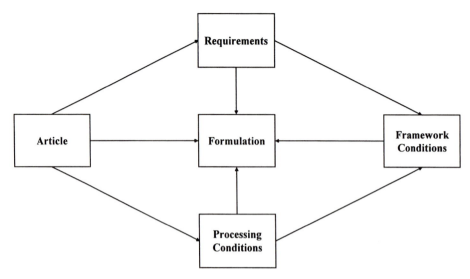

Figure 8.13   Structure of TEXPERTO as described by Frie and Poppenwimmer (1992)

for the formulation (e.g. article is weak in formaldehyde). In the search for a suitable formulation, TEXPERTO only selected ingredients which took all the set framework conditions into consideration, observed all restrictions and which were compatible with each other. If problems occurred, the system informed the user of the difficulties and interacted with the user to reach a satisfactory decision.

In addition to the selection of ingredients, the system calculated both quantities and solution concentrations for the process. Depending on the size of the charge and the solution uptake of the articles, the system also calculated the consumption of the solution as well as the total quantities of the ingredients. Data on the solution and its dilution could also be derived. This was necessary to avoid the occurrence of problems. A database of technical information on all the ingredients was available within TEXPERTO to provide the user with details of the ingredients used in the formulation.

TEXPERTO provided, as its output, a detailed overview of the formulation including all processing steps and, if need be, a list of expected problems. Unfortunately no technical details of the system were given, nor any details of its usage. However, the authors did make a comment that the system did fulfil all expectations and provided customer service personnel with readily available specialist knowledge enabling them to deal with enquiries with consistency and certainty (Frie and Poppenwimmer, 1992).

8.9   Vinyl Coatings

Flexible polyvinyl chloride (PVC) compounds are used extensively for floor and wall coverings. Formulations include plasticisers, stabilisers, diluents and pigments to give the desired properties of rigidity and flexibility. Blowing agents, which cause the formulation to expand into a foam when heated in an oven, can also be added to create vinyl foams. These so-called cellular vinyls exhibit high tensile and tear properties, good abrasion resistance, good chemical resistance, good ageing characteristics and excellent dimensional stability and are ideal for floor and wall coverings. Using the prototype formulation kernel developed as part of the UK Alvey Programme in 1987 (i.e. the forerunner of PFES), personnel at Schering Industrial Products Ltd UK and Logica UK Ltd developed a public demonstrator based on the formulation of foams using the GENITRON range of blowing agents produced by Schering. The company provided a number of technical services to customers who used blowing agents in their formulations and the system developed mimicked the generation of a formulation based on the GENITRON range of products which would satisfy the application requirements of a customer.

Initially the user was asked to specify the problem to be solved: the process parameters by which the formulation would be made (e.g. oven temperature, oven dwell time, etc.); the required performance parameters of the final formulation (e.g. expansion factor, viscosity characteristics, etc.); and information regarding the end use of the product and any user preferences. The system then decided on the components to be used in the formulation, displaying each chosen component one at a time to allow the user to accept or reject the decision. Levels of each ingredient were set to produce a paper formulation. The user was then asked to subject the formulation to a variety of tests and enter the results. The system attempted to reformulate by either changing the polyvinyl chloride or altering the levels of the ingredients. The task structure representative of this type of formulation is shown in Figure 8.14. For a full description of this system together with a full listing of the rules the reader is referred to Volume 4 of the Alvey Project Report (1987).

The system was developed to demonstrate the practicality of building a formulation expert system using the prototype formulation kernel. It included most facets of the architecture of the kernel and embodied a reasonably complete breadth of knowledge used in formulating vinyl coatings. It was able to generate realistic and accurate formulations for some classes of the formulation domain.

8.10   Vinyl Pipes

In addition to coatings, polyvinyl chloride is also used in the manufacture of rigid pipes. For these formulations it is necessary to add heat stabilisers (approx. 2%), lubricants (approx. 3%), processing aids (approx. 3%), and, to impart rigidity and strength, impact modifiers (approx. 15%), and fillers and pigments (approx. 30%). The specific additives and their concentrations used depend on the requirements of the product. For instance, an underground pipe for potable water would require non-toxic, non-migrating additives and the underground deployment demands high impact strength, compression and abrasion resistance. It is the task of the formulator to translate the many requirements demanded by the final use and manufacturing equipment into technical variables, e.g. final appearance to melt flow index, bursting pressure of a pressurised pipe into yield strength, and flexural resistance into modulus of elasticity, and to optimise the inherent attributes of the polymer and additives by varying their respective concentrations to achieve the desired characteristic.

Such an application has recently been developed by personnel at a consultancy company (Investigacion y Desarrollo CA) working under contract for a plastics company (Plasticos Petroquimica CA) in Maracaibo, Venezuela (Quintero-Arcaya *et al.*, 1995). The system, appropriately named Formulator, combined two databases, one specifically designed to contain all the knowledge on the additives used in the application, the other an interactive encyclopaedia of polymers with access

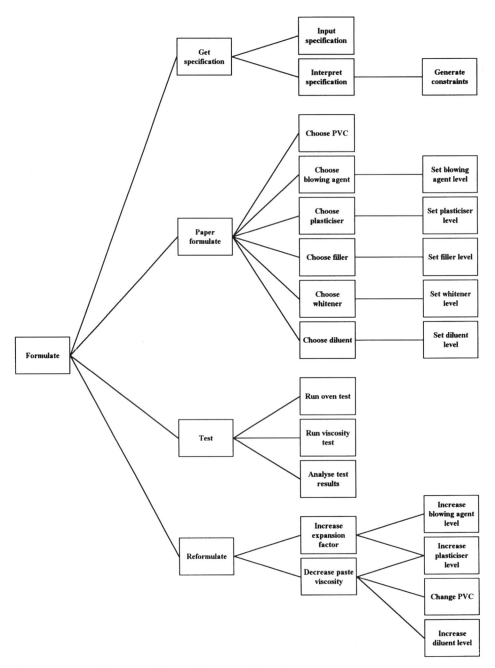

Figure 8.14 Task structure for vinyl covering formulation

to technical concepts and machine drawings (Figure 8.15). Formulation requirements were divided into those demanded by the final use of the pipes, e.g. transported liquid, wall thickness, outside diameter, impact strength, etc. and those demanded by the manufacturing equipment, e.g. single or double screw extruder, counter or co-rotating screws, etc. An inference engine then made the transformation of the requirement into property and characteristics and navigated between the additive

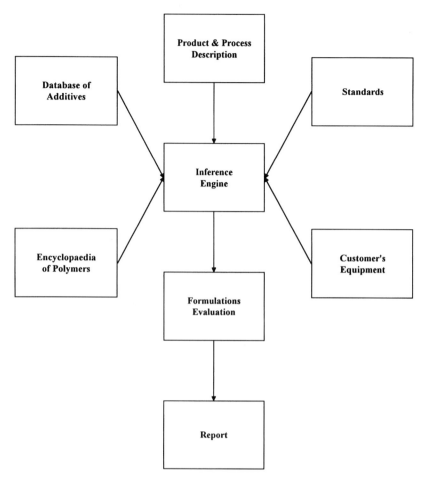

Figure 8.15 Structure of the expert system described by Quintero-Arcaya *et al.* (1995) for formulating vinyl pipes

and property space to obtain the desired formulations. The final outcome was a set of formulations that fitted the multiple constraints imposed by the requirements. The system also contained a module appropriately called the Formulation Evaluator which examined a given formulation and compared it with those recommended by the system both quantitatively and in terms of performance.

Unfortunately no further details of the system architecture or usage were given in the paper. However, the authors claim that the system was not limited to the formulation of pipes produced from polyvinyl chloride but could be easily extended to other thermoplastics and applications. The authors also claimed that, to the best of their knowledge, it was the first application of expert systems in the field of polyvinyl chloride formulation.

8.11 Wool Dyeing

Wool dyeing is a complex operation. Various pre- and post-processing operations (e.g. bleaching, carbonising, chemical fixing) are necessary which not only determine

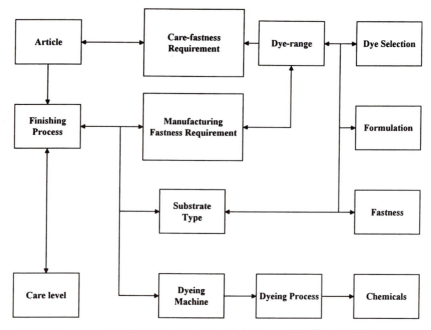

Figure 8.16   Structure of WOOLY as described by Frie and Walliser (1988)

the quality of the end product (e.g. fastness, physical properties of the wool) but also influence the selection of the dyestuff. In addition to the quality of the wool, the dyeing machine as well as the specific requests of the customer often require a special selection of dyes and an adapted dyeing process.

Figure 8.16 illustrates the interaction of the various factors in the wool dyeing process and forms the structure of WOOLY, an expert system designed by Frie and Walliser (1988) of Sandoz (now Clariant) in Switzerland. The user entered which woollen article was to be processed together with the care-fastness require-ment (dry-cleaning only, hand washable or machine washable). This resulted in the production of a care-fastness profile which comprised all the requirements demanded of such an article. WOOLY actually contained a database of profiles for a large number of woollen articles corresponding to those given by the International Wool Secretariat. Special profiles could be entered at any time.

From the profile, WOOLY generated a standard finishing process which the user could adapt or modify. Once agreed WOOLY listed the manufacturing fast-ness requirements necessary to determine the choice of the dyestuffs. WOOLY always recommended the dye range which just fulfilled the requirements based on the assumption that the greater the wet strength of a dyestuff, the more difficult it was to use for dyeing. Formulation of the dyestuff was selected using colour cards and the fastness of the formulation was calculated. After it had been established that the selected formulation fulfilled the demanded fastness requirement, WOOLY searched for a suitable dyeing process and dyeing machine. A temperature/time profile for the dyeing process was also created.

No technical details on this expert system exist in the literature and hence it is difficult to assess its complexity. The authors gave no indication of its usage although they did comment that such a system would not replace experts in the domain.

8.12   Szechwan Cooking

Although not strictly product formulation, the creation of a new recipe in cooking exhibits characteristics of the formulation process. Hence, when considering the applications of expert systems in formulation, it is pertinent to review those developed for cooking. Of specific importance is CHEF, a case-based reasoning system (as opposed to the rule-based reasoning used for all previous applications) that creates new Szechwan recipes based on the user's requests out of its memory of old ones (Hammond, 1986, 1989). Szechwan cooking is characterised by the use of hot chilli peppers indigenous to the region combined with aromatic spices (e.g. ginger).

An overview of the structure of CHEF is shown in Figure 8.17. Basically it consisted of six modules with a simulator. The input to CHEF was a set of requirements for different tastes, textures, ingredients and types of dishes. These were sent to the ANTICIPATOR module which anticipated any problems that might arise based on past failures and predicted any problems that would have to be avoided. The requirements now as goals and predictions were then passed to the RETRIEVER module. This searched for a recipe in memory that best satisfied the requirements and avoided any of the predicted problems. In searching for the best match this module used three kinds of knowledge:

- Memory of recipes indexed by the requirements satisfied and the problems avoided.

- A similarity measure allowing it to determine partial matches.

- A value hierarchy allowing it to judge the relative importance of the requirements to be achieved.

The result from these was a past recipe that matched some if not all of the requirements. This best matched recipe was then sent to a MODIFIER module which altered it to satisfy any of the input requirements that were not already achieved. This was accomplished using modification rules which were descriptors of the steps that were to be added or deleted from existing recipes in order to make them satisfy new requirements. Along with these rules was a set of critics and specifications that looked at the recipe and, on the basis of the ingredients involved, corrected difficulties that had been associated with them in the past.

Once the modified recipe had been completed it was run in the simulator module using a set of causal rules. At the end of the simulation, CHEF checked whether all the requirements had been achieved. If positive the recipe was then sent to the STORER module indexed by the requirements it achieved and the problems it avoided. If the recipe failed either because a desired requirement had not been achieved or an undesired state had been achieved (i.e. the vegetables had gone soggy) it was sent to the REPAIRER module. Here the characterisation of the failure was built using two types of knowledge: a vocabulary for describing failures; and a set of repair strategies that corresponded to these descriptors. The recipe was revised using the required repair strategy and sent to the STORER module indexed by the requirements achieved and the problem(s) avoided.

In order to learn from failure, CHEF used an ASSIGNER module to look at the failed recipe and decide what features would be predictive if that failure occurred in the future (e.g. the iodine taste of stir-fried fish, duck fat, excess liquid

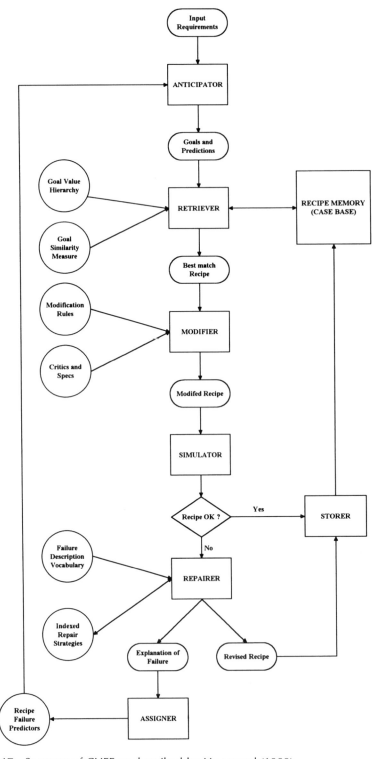

Figure 8.17 Structure of CHEF as described by Hammond (1989)

in soufflés). These were then sent back to the ANTICIPATOR module for future reference. The power of CHEF was directly dependent on its ability to reuse recipes and the only way to reuse recipes effectively was to take seriously the concept of learning to anticipate failures and search for recipes that avoid problems. While the original CHEF was to demonstrate case-based reasoning rather than develop a new cookery book, CHEF did create new recipes. Working from an initial base of ten recipes obtained from available books on Szechwan cooking, it created 21 new recipes on the basis of users' requirements. For a full description of CHEF the reader is referred to Hammond's book on case-based planning (Hammond, 1989).

Hammond *et al.* (1996) have recently proposed an extension of CHEF. Appropriately named CYBER CHEF, it has been designed to read requests posted to the rec.food.recipes newsgroup on the Internet and respond with recipes based on the group's own archive. CYBER CHEF will perform all the same functions as CHEF but with a larger case library taken from various on-line recipe archives. Ultimately it is intended that CYBER CHEF will react to input requests in natural language, retrieve and possibly modify recipes from the case library. To replace the simulator program in CHEF, CYBER CHEF will receive feedback from newsgroup readers who have tried the recipes. Currently the implementation only deals with recipes for sauces and can only retrieve but not modify recipes from the library (Hammond *et al.*, 1996).

8.13 Conclusion

Applications of product formulation expert systems are now widespread. Many have progressed from the prototype stage through to working systems complementing the decision making of formulators. The impact and benefits as well as the issues surrounding their implementation will be discussed in Chapters 11 and 12 respectively.

References

ALVEY PROJECT REPORT, 1987, IKBS/052, *Product Formulation Expert System*, Vol. 2, Description of Applications; Vol. 4, The Public Demonstrator, London: DTI.

BASSEMIR, R.W., BEAN, O., WASILEWSKI, O., KLINE, D., HILLIS, W., SU, C., STEEL, I.R. and RUSTERHOLZ, W.E., 1995, Inks, in KROSCHWITZ, J.I. and HOWE-GRANT, M. (eds), *Kirk-Othmer Encyclopedia of Chemical Technology*, Vol. 14, 4th edition, pp. 482–503, New York: Wiley-Interscience.

BOOSER, E.R., 1995, Lubrication and lubricants, in KROSCHWITZ, J.I. and HOWE-GRANT, M. (eds), *Kirk-Othmer Encyclopedia of Chemical Technology*, Vol. 15, 4th edition, pp. 463–517, New York: Wiley-Interscience.

FRIE, G. and POPPENWIMMER, K., 1992, TEXPERTO – ein expertensystem fur die ausrustung, *Textilveredlung*, **27**, 276–279.

FRIE, G. and WALLISER, R., 1988, WOOLY – ein expertensystem fur den wollfarber, *Textilveredlung*, **23**, 203–205.

FRISCH, P.D., LALKA, G.J. and ORRICK, J.F., 1990, INFORM – a generalised ink formulation assistant, *American Ink Maker*, **68** (10), 56–68.

GUPTA, T. and GHOSH, B.K., 1988, A survey of expert systems in manufacturing and process planning, *Computers in Industry*, **11**, 195–204.

HAMMOND, K.J., 1986, CHEF: a model of case-based planning, *Proceedings of Fifth National Conference on Artificial Intelligence*, pp. 267–271, Menlo Park, CA: AAAI Press.

HAMMOND, K.J., 1989, *Case-based planning – viewing planning as a memory task*, San Diego, CA: Academic Press.

HAMMOND, K.J., Burke, R. and SCHMITT, K., 1996, A case-based approach to knowledge navigation, in LEAKE, D.B. (ed.), *Cased-based Reasoning, Experiences, Lessons and Future Directions*, pp. 125–136, Menlo Park, CA: AAAI Press.

HOHNE, B.A. and HOUGHTON, R.D., 1986, An expert system for the formulation of agricultural chemicals, in PIERCE, T.H. and HOHNE, B.A. (eds), *Artificial Intelligence Applications in Chemistry*, ACS Symposium series 306, pp. 87–97, Chicago: American Chemical Society.

LINDNER, V., 1993, Propellants, in KROSCHWITZ, J.I. and HOWE-GRANT, M. (eds), *Kirk-Othmer Encyclopedia of Chemical Technology*, Vol. 10, 4th edition, pp. 69–125, New York: Wiley-Interscience.

LUNN, K., ARCHIBALD, I.G., REDFEARN, J.J., ROBINSON, A., BAMIGBOYE, A., COPE, M.D. and HIRD, B.T., 1991, An expert system for formulating lubricating oils, *A.I. in Engineering*, **6**, 74–85.

QUINTERO-ARCAYA, R.A., MARTINEZ, R., CASTILLO, M.M., PACHECO, C., MORALES, I., RUIZ, C.E. and HAOR, M., 1995, Formulator: formulating PVC for pipes – an artificial intelligence approach, *Annu. Tech. Conf. Soc. Plast. Eng.*, **53** (3), 3569–3573.

RYCHENER, M.D., FARINACCI, M.L., HULTHAGE, I. and Fox, M.S., 1985, Integration of multiple knowledge sources in ALADIN, an alloy design system, *IEEE J. Engng.*, 878–882.

SHAW, F.J. and FIFER, R.A., 1988, *A Preliminary Report on Developing an Expert System for Computer-aided Formulation of Propellants*, BRL-TR-2895, US Army Ballistic Research Laboratory.

SMITH, A., 1995, *Future Trends in Pesticide Formulation*, AGROW Report No. DS 92, Richmond, Surrey: PJB Publications.

STALEY, J.T. and HAUPIN, W., 1992, Aluminium and aluminium alloys, in KROSCHWITZ, J.I. and HOWE-GRANT, M. (eds), *Kirk-Othmer Encyclopedia of Chemical Technology*, Vol. 2, 4th edition, pp. 184–251, New York: Wiley-Interscience.

STONE, E., 1987, Resin and varnish formulation, *American Ink Maker*, **65** (12), 26–36 and 72–74.

VAIL, D.L., 1983, Textiles (finishing), in GRAYSON, M. and ECKROTH, D. (eds), *Kirk-Othmer Encyclopedia of Chemical Technology*, Vol. 22, 3rd edition, pp. 769–802, New York: Wiley-Interscience.

WOOD, M., 1991, Expert systems save formulation time, *Lab-Equipment Digest*, December, 17–19.

9

Applications of Expert Systems – Pharmaceutical

9.1 Introduction

Pharmaceutical formulation is the process by which a chemical entity (i.e. a drug) is converted into an effective, safe, stable and convenient to use medicine. There are many formulation types depending on the route of administration of the active ingredient:

- **Capsules** – These are solid preparations primarily intended for oral administration with hard or soft shells comprised of gelatin and small amounts of other ingredients such as plasticisers, opaque fillers and colouring agents. The contents may be powders, liquids or pastes formulated so as to cause no deterioration of the shell. Powder formulations consist of one or more active ingredients mixed with a diluent or filler, a disintegrant, a lubricant and possibly a surface active agent. The powders can be granulated with a binding agent to improve flow and uniformity of weight. Powders are generally filled into hard shells while liquids are filled directly into soft shells. Suspensions and pastes of sufficiently high viscosity can be filled into both types of shell. With liquid or suspension formulations in soft shells, partial migration of the capsule contents and shell constituents may occur because of the nature of the materials and the surfaces in contact.

    All capsules have to comply with limits for uniformity of weight and content of the active ingredient, disintegration (break up in solution) and dissolution of the active ingredient.

- **Oral liquids** – These consist of solutions, suspensions or emulsion of one or more active ingredients mixed with preservatives, antioxidants, dispersing agents, suspending agents, thickeners, emulsifiers, solubilisers, wetting agents, colours and flavourings in a suitable vehicle, generally water. They may be supplied ready for use or may be prepared before use from concentrated liquid preparations or from granules or powders by the addition of the vehicle. Suspensions and emulsions may separate on standing and may require re-dispersing by shaking before use but all preparations must remain sufficiently stable to enable a homogeneous dose to be withdrawn.

All preparations have to comply with limits for uniformity of content and dose.

- **Tablets** – These are solid preparations, each containing a single dose of one or more active ingredients mixed with a filler/diluent, a disintegrant, a binder, a surfactant, a glidant, a lubricant and possibly colorants and flavourings. Tablets are prepared by compacting the powders in a punch and die and can exist in a variety of shapes (round, oval, oblong, triangular, etc.), sizes and weights dependent on the amount (dose) of active ingredient and the intended method of administration (swallowable, dissolved in water, inserted under the tongue, chewable, etc.). Tablets also provide a broad range of drug release responses ranging from rapid release providing fast relief of symptoms, to a modified release over a period of 8–12 hours, maintaining adequate control of symptoms with the convenience of a single administration. Tablets may also be coated with either sugar or a thin polymer film.

  Tablets have to comply with limits on uniformity of weight and content of the active ingredient, strength, disintegration and dissolution of all the active ingredients.

- **Parenterals** – These are sterile preparations intended for administration by injection, infusion or implantation. Injections are sterile solutions, emulsions or suspensions prepared by dissolving, emulsifying or suspending the active ingredient together with suitable pH adjusters, tonicity adjusters, solubilisers, antioxidants, chelating agents and antimicrobial preservatives in appropriate concentrations in Water for Injection, a suitable non-aqueous liquid or a mixture of the two. If there are stability problems, the formulation can be prepared as a freeze dried sterile powder to which the appropriate sterile vehicle is added prior to use. Formulations that cannot be sterilised in their final containers must be prepared using aseptic techniques. Preparations can be single dose or multi-dose, supplied in glass ampoules, bottles, vials or prefilled syringes.

  Infusions, or more correctly intravenous infusions, are sterile aqueous solutions or emulsions intended for administration in large volume.

  Implants or sterile solid preparations of a size and shape for implantation are designed to release their active ingredient over an extended period of time. They are presented individually using specially designed syringes.

  All parenteral preparations have to comply with regulations on sterility, pyrogens and uniformity of content.

- **Topicals** – Topicals are semi-solid preparations e.g. creams, ointments and gels intended to be applied to the skin or to certain mucous surfaces for local action, percutaneous penetration of the active ingredient, protective action or as an emollient. Preparations may be single or multi-phase, containing one or more active ingredients formulated to be miscible, immiscible or emulsifiable with the skin secretion. All types of preparations can be categorised as being hydrophilic or hydrophobic. Hydrophilic creams contain water as the continuous phase with oil-in-water emulsifying agents such as triethanolamine soaps and polysorbates combined with water-in-oil emulsifying agents such as monoglycerides and sorbitan esters. Hydrophobic creams have the lipophilic phase as the continuous phase with water-in-oil emulsifying agents. Hydrophobic gels (known as oleogels) are based on liquid paraffin or fatty oils gelled with colloidal silica or aluminium or zinc soaps. Hydrophilic gels consist of water, glycerol or propylene glycol with cellulose derivatives or carboxyvinyl polymers as gelling agents. Hydrophobic ointments use hard, soft and liquid paraffins, vegetable oils, fats and waxes while hydrophilic ointments use mixtures of liquid and solid polyethylene glycols.

All preparations have to comply with regulations for sterility (if required) and storage/stability.

■ **Eye preparations** – These are preparations specifically intended for administration to the eye in the form of drops, lotions and ointments. Eye drops are sterile aqueous or oily solutions or suspensions of one or more active ingredients containing tonicity, viscosity and pH adjusters, solubilisers, antioxidants and antimicrobial preservatives intended for administration into the eye as drops. Eye lotions are sterile aqueous liquids of similar formulation intended for washing or bathing the eye. Eye ointments are sterile, semi-solid formulations intended for application to the conjunctiva.

All preparations must comply with regulations for sterility and stability and be formulated to minimise irritation.

■ **Suppositories and pessaries** – These are solid preparations containing one or more active ingredients dissolved or dispersed in a suitable base which may be either dispersible in water or melt at body temperature. Suppositories are intended for rectal administration, pessaries are intended for vaginal administration.

Both types of preparation must comply with limits for uniformity of weight and active ingredient content, disintegration and dissolution of the active ingredient.

■ **Inhalation preparations** – Inhalation preparations can be solutions, suspensions or powders intended to be inhaled as aerosols for administration to the lung. They can be supplied as metered dose pressurised aerosols, solution nebulisers or dry powder inhalers in various designs. In all cases the size of the particles or droplets to be inhaled should be controlled to localise their deposition in the required target area of the respiratory tract.

In addition to those mentioned other formulations used in pharmacy include liniments, lotions, pastes, paints and extracts. A distribution of formulation types for pharmaceutical preparations manufactured in the UK for the period 1985–1986 is shown in Figure 9.1 (Wells, 1988). It can be seen that oral preparations in the form of tablets, capsules and liquids account for nearly 75 per cent of the total, with tablets being by far the most used formulation type. Although these data are some ten years old, experience has indicated that the distribution shown in Figure 9.1 is unlikely to have changed significantly.

For all formulations the correct choice of additives or excipients is paramount in the provision of efficacy, stability and safety. For instance, excipients may be chemically or physically incompatible with the active ingredient or they may exhibit batchwise variability to such an extent that at the extremes of the specification the formulation may fail to release the active ingredient. In addition some excipients may promote irritation when the formulation is administered, while others may cause dust explosions under specific conditions of manufacture. Hence it is not surprising that this domain has been a productive one for expert systems.

The first recorded reference to the use of expert systems in pharmaceutical product formulation was by Bradshaw on 27 April 1989 in the London *Financial Times* (Bradshaw, 1989) closely followed by an article in the autumn of the same year by Walko (1989). Both refer to the work then being undertaken by personnel at ICI (now Zeneca) Pharmaceuticals, UK and Logica UK Ltd to develop expert

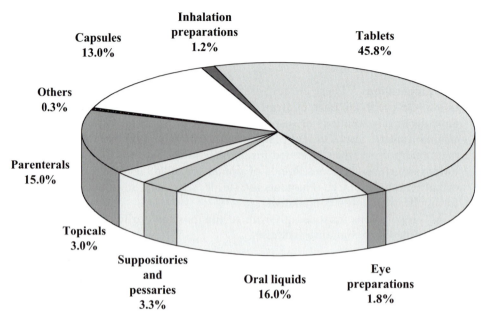

Figure 9.1 Distribution by number of formulation types for pharmaceuticals in the UK for the period 1985–1986 (Wells, 1988)

systems for formulating pharmaceuticals using PFES (Chapter 3). Since that time several companies and academic institutions have reported on their experiences in this area. In this chapter published applications on tablets, capsules and parenterals are reviewed, not under application areas as in Chapter 8, but under company or institution name.

9.2   The Cadila System

Cadila Laboratories Ltd of Ahmedabad, India has developed an expert system for the formulation of tablets for active ingredients based on their physical, chemical and biological properties (Ramani *et al.*, 1992). The system first identifies the desirable properties in the excipients for optimum compatibility with the active ingredient and then selects those that have the required properties based on the assumption that all tablet formulations comprise at least one binder, one disintegrant and one lubricant. Other excipients such as diluents (fillers) or glidants are then added as required.

Knowledge was acquired through 'active collaboration' with domain experts over a period of six to seven months. It is structured in two knowledge bases in a spreadsheet format. In the knowledge base concerning the interactions between active ingredients and excipients, the columns represent the properties of the excipients with descriptors of 'strong', 'moderate' and 'weak' and the rows represent the properties of the active ingredients e.g. functional groups (primary amines, secondary amines, highly acidic, etc.), solubility (very soluble, freely soluble, soluble, sparingly soluble, slightly soluble, very slightly soluble, insoluble), density (low, moderate, high) etc. Each cell in the spreadsheet then represents the knowledge of the interaction between the various properties. Production rules derived from this knowledge are of the form:

IF (functional group of active ingredient is 'primary/secondary amine')

THEN (add 'strong' binder)

AND (add 'strong' disintegrant)

AND (avoid lactose)

or:

IF (functional group of active ingredient is 'highly acidic')

THEN (add 'moderate' binder)

AND (add 'moderate' disintegrant)

AND (avoid starch)

or:

IF (active ingredient is soluble)

THEN (add 'weak' binder)

AND (add 'weak' disintegrant)

A similar approach is used for the knowledge base concerning the excipients where the columns now represent details (e.g. name, minimum, maximum and normal concentrations) of the excipients and the rows their properties (e.g. type and the descriptors – strong, moderate and weak). Each cell in the spreadsheet then represents the name and the amount to be added to the formulation.

The system written in PROLOG is menu driven and interactive with the user. The user is first prompted to input all the known properties of the new active ingredient. Where the properties have descriptors, these are displayed for selection by the user. All information can be edited to correct errors. The expert system then consults the knowledge bases suggesting compatible excipients and a formulation. If the latter is unacceptable, the system provides alternative formulations with explanations. All formulations can be stored along with explanations if necessary. The user is able to update the knowledge base via an interface with a spreadsheet. An example of a formulation generated for the analgesic drug paracetamol or acetominophen (dose 500 mg) is shown in Table 9.1. It is interesting to note that the diluent/filler is unnamed; it can be assumed that it will not be lactose since the relevant production rule indicates that there would be an interaction with the secondary amine in paracetamol. Furthermore, an examination of formulations on the market indicates that none contain lactose and that some contain mixtures of maize starch, sodium starch glycolate, stearic acid, magnesium stearate and microcrystalline cellulose, adding further weight to the choice by the Cadila system.

The prototype system when first implemented had 150 rules but this has been rapidly expanded to approximately 300 rules to increase reliability. It is expected that it will evolve further over time. The system is regarded as being highly successful, providing competitive advantage to the company (Ramani *et al.*, 1992).

9.3 The Galenical Development System, Heidelberg

This system, with the abbreviation GSH, has been developed by personnel in the Department of Pharmaceutics and Biopharmaceutics and the Department of Medical Informatics at the University of Heidelberg, Germany. It has been designed

Table 9.1   An example of a tablet formulation for the analgesic drug paracetamol as generated by the Cadila system (Ramani *et al.*, 1992)

Input		
Dose	500 mg	
Functional group	Secondary amines	
Solubility	Sparingly soluble	
Density	Moderate	
Hygroscopicity	Moderate	
Dissolution	Slow	
Desired tablet weight	570 mg	
Output		
Active agent	Paracetamol	500.0 mg
Binder	Pregelatinised starch	43.7 mg
Disintegrant	Sodium starch glycolate	5.0 mg
Lubricant	Stearic acid	2.5 mg
Diluent/filler	Unnamed	20.0 mg
	Tablet weight	571.2 mg

to provide assistance in the development of a range of formulations starting from the chemical and physical properties of an active ingredient. The project was initiated in 1990 under the direction of Stricker (Stricker *et al.*, 1991) and the system has been extensively revised and enhanced in the interim (Stricker *et al.*, 1994; Frank *et al.*, 1997). Originally implemented using object oriented C on an IBM 6150 workstation, the system has recently been upgraded using SMALLTALK V running under the Windows operating system on a 486 processor with at least 8MB RAM.

Various forms of knowledge representation are used depending on the type of knowledge. Knowledge about objects (e.g. functional groups in the active ingredient, excipients, processes, etc.) as well as their properties and relationships is represented in frames using an object oriented approach. Causal relationships are represented as rules, functional connections as formulas and procedural knowledge as algorithms. The system currently has knowledge bases for aerosols, intravenous injection solutions, capsules (hard shell powder) and tablets (direct compression), each incorporating information on all aspects of that dosage formulation (e.g. properties of the excipients to be added, compatibility, processing operations, packaging and containers and storage conditions) with each aspect being given a reliability factor (*Sicherheitsfaktor*) to indicate its accuracy/reliability. Values for each factor varied between 0 and 9 in the original version of the system (Stricker *et al.*, 1991) but, in later versions, values between 0 and 1 are used. The values are propagated using the arithmetic minimum rule and are not used for any decisions. They only serve as indicators of the accuracy/reliability of the knowledge.

The approach used in the system is the decomposition of the overall process into individual distinct development steps, each step focusing on one problem associated with a subset of its specifications or constraints for the formulation. A problem is considered solved if its predicted outcome satisfies its associated constraints. The problems are worked through in succession, care being taken that any solution should not violate any constraints from previous steps. For simplicity the developers imposed a predefined ordering onto the development steps, providing a back-tracking mechanism to go back to a previous step or abort. This ordering minimises dependency between development steps which might result in an action causing a constraint previously satisfied to be violated. It also reduces the complexity of the problem to be solved.

The procedural model for one development step (e.g. for the choice of an excipient) is shown in Figure 9.2. In any development step the first decision is whether or not to proceed with any actions since the problem may have already been solved in previous steps. This is done by comparing the predicted or relevant properties of the current formulation with the initial specification. If the answer is negative then further action is required, if positive the problem has been solved. Once this has been decided actions need to be defined and ranked. Knowledge for this is by means of hierarchically structural rule sets to form a decision tree where each leaf node consists of a subgroup of actions and each branch a rule. The rules in a rule set are ordered as the simplest and most straightforward way of handling conflict. Ranking numbers are used as the basis for the selection strategy, the concept being to search for the best alternative in terms of the highest score, these being the sum of the values of the constants to be resolved within the development step (e.g. solubility, compressibility, etc.) and their weights indicating their respective importance (Frank *et al.*, 1997). It should be noted that this method of ranking is different from that used originally by Stricker *et al.* (1991), where the lowest score was regarded as the best alternative.

Once the action is selected, the decision is checked in terms of whether or not the measure has adverse effects on the active ingredient in terms of physical or chemical incompatibility. This does not necessarily mean a rejection of the action since knowledge on compatibilities is generally of a qualitative nature with little quantification to denote severity. Hence the overall decision is left to the user.

Calculation of the amounts of excipients is by the use of formulae with a rule-based mechanism for selecting the appropriate formula. A rule-based mechanism is also used to determine the appropriate function for predicting the property of the intermediate formulation. This is necessary for checking whether or not the original specifications have been satisfied and the action is successful. If negative, the chosen action is rejected and the next action in the ranking is tried. It is possible that none of the ranked actions are successful. If this is the case then knowledge-based back-tracking is used to determine which of the previous development steps to return to. Usually background pharmaceutical knowledge is applied to determine why the current development step was unsuccessful and a development step chosen that can solve the root cause of the problem.

In any expert system, explanations of the decisions made are important both for instruction of the user and for maintenance of the system. Explanations in GSH take several forms. There are explanations for the development steps and their ordering provided by the designer of the knowledge base. Detailed explanations of the rules activated, formulae used or individual scores of actions can be generated if required and canned text and literature references are provided for general knowledge.

A simplified task structure for generating an intravenous injection solution is shown in Figure 9.3. The input to the system includes all the known properties of the active ingredient requiring to be formulated (e.g. solubility, stability, impurities, pKa, presence/absence of functional groups, etc.) with user defined labels relating the specific drug property to the required product property. Use of the

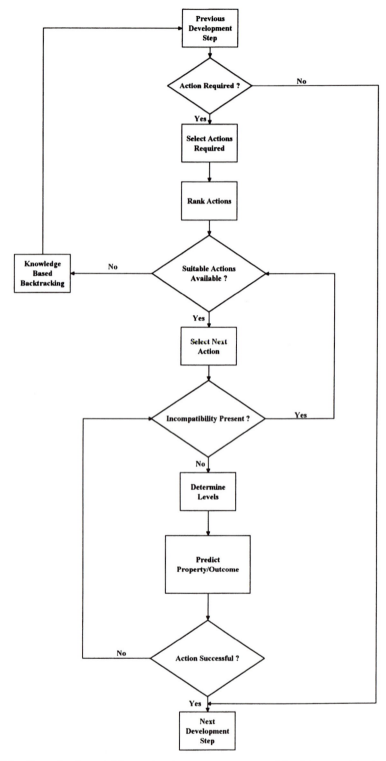

Figure 9.2 Procedural model for a development step as used in GSH (modified after Frank *et al.*, 1997)

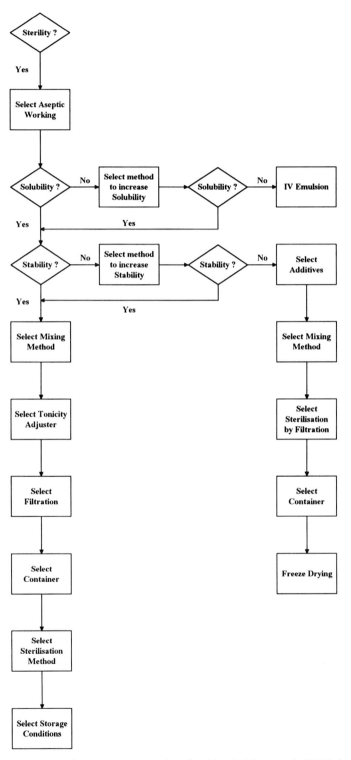

Figure 9.3 Structure of the expert system described by Stricker *et al.* (1991) for the formulation of intravenous injection solutions

Table 9.2 An example of an intravenous injection solution formulation for the cardiac drug digoxin as generated by GSH (Stricker *et al.*, 1994)

Formulation

Active	Digoxin	0.1 mg
Solvent 1	1,2-Propandiol	0.5 ml
	Water for Injection to	1.0 ml

Packaging
Brown glass ampoules

Product properties

Property	Specification	Actual	RF*
Active (mg)	0.095	0.098	1.0
Volume (ml)	1.0	1.0	1.0
pH	3–9	7.0	1.0
Freezing point depression (°C)	0.5–20	13.2	0.8
Shelf life at 25°C (years)	≥ 3	5.0	1.0
Decomposition at 25°C (mol)	≤ 3	1.8	0.7

* RF, reliability factor

Table 9.3 An example of a hard gelatin capsule formulation for the antifungal drug griseofulvin as generated by GSH (Frank *et al.*, 1997)

Formulation

Active	Griseofulvin	150.0 mg
Diluent	Microcrystalline cellulose (PH102)	199.2 mg
Lubricant	Magnesium stearate	3.5 mg

Production process
High shear mixer for deagglomeration, premix and main mix
Add lubricant, Planetary mixer at 12 rpm for three minutes
Capsule filling machine type 1

Packaging
Foil blisters (PVC and aluminium foil)

system results in the production of four packages: product formulation; production method; recommended packaging and storage conditions; and predicted product properties. All the outputs are provided with reliability factors. An example for an intravenous injection solution of the cardiac drug digoxin is shown in Table 9.2 and an example for a hard gelatin capsule of the antifungal drug griseofulvin is shown in Table 9.3. Comparison of a 0.1 mg commercial formulation of digoxin with that shown in Table 9.2 indicates that the same co-solvent is used (1,2-propandiol, presumably to enhance solubility) and ethanol. However the commercial formulation is more sophisticated since it also contains buffer (disodium hydrogen phosphate/ citric acid).

At present, knowledge bases for aerosols, intravenous injection solutions, hard gelatin capsules and direct compression tablets have been completed and a further four for coated forms, granules, freeze dried formulations and pellets are in different stages of development. Trials have demonstrated that the system proposes formulations that are acceptable to formulators and in December 1996, the system was first introduced for field trials in a pharmaceutical company.

9.4 The University of London/Capsugel System

This system, developed as part of a PhD programme by Lai, Podczeck and Newton at the School of Pharmacy, University of London, supported by Daumesnil of Capsugel, Switzerland together with personnel from the University of Kyoto, Japan and the University of Maryland, USA is designed to aid the formulation of hard gelatin capsules (Lai *et al.*, 1995, 1996). The system (Figure 9.4) is unique in that its knowledge base is broad containing:

- A database of literature references associated with the formulation of hard gelatin capsules which is frequently updated through monitoring of current literature.

- Information on excipients used and their properties. This database currently contains information on 72 excipients and is frequently updated. Data can be retrieved via a menu.

- An analysis of marketed formulations from Germany, Italy, Belgium, France and the USA. This is used to identify trends in formulation and identify guidelines on the use of excipients. Currently the database contains information on 750 formulations of 250 active ingredients. It is frequently updated and data can be retrieved via a menu.

- Experience and non-proprietary knowledge obtained over a period of 18 months from a group of industrial experts from Europe, USA and Japan.

- Results from statistically designed experiments identifying factors which influence the filling and *in-vitro* release performance of model active ingredients.

The system uses production rules with a decision tree implemented in C, coupled with a user interface through which the user can both access the databases and develop new formulations. To assist in collecting all necessary input data, a questionnaire has been designed. Called the expert system input package it requires information on the physical properties of the active ingredient (e.g. dose, particle shape, particle size, solubility, wettability, adhesion to metal surfaces, melting point and bulk density); compatibility of the active ingredient with excipients (e.g. fillers/diluents, disintegrants, lubricants, glidants and surfactants); and properties of excipients used by the user and manufacturing conditions (e.g. capsule sizes, fill weights, densification techniques, granulation techniques) used by the user.

From these data the system uses a variety of methods to evaluate and predict properties of mixtures of the active ingredient and the excipients. For instance it uses Carr's compressibility index (Carr, 1965) to predict the flow properties which are used to give an indication of the ability to produce a uniform blend and the Kawakita equation (Ludde and Kawakita, 1966) to predict a maximum in the volume reduction of the powder achievable by the application of low pressure. The packing properties are obviously important to give the volume that a given weight

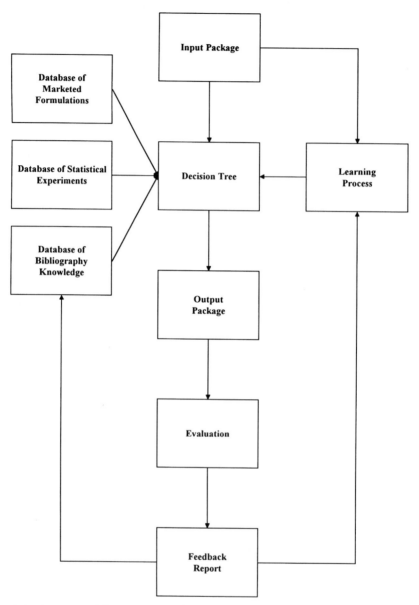

Figure 9.4 Structure of the University of London/Capsugel system as described by Lai *et al.* (1995, 1996)

of powder occupies to indicate the size of capsule shell that can be used. When wet granulation is offered as the preferred method of densification, the system only offers advice on the choice of a granulating liquid and binder; no choice on the granulation procedure is offered.

The system provides an output package which includes a formulation with any necessary powder processing and filling conditions, the required capsule size, a statistical design to optimise the formulation quantitatively, specification of excipients used, recommended tests to validate the formulation and a complete documentation of the decision process.

An interesting addition to the system is a semi-automatic learning tool. This monitors user habits and collects data about the use of excipients. Statistical analysis is performed on these data allowing agreed alterations to be made to the database. The user is also asked to reply to a questionnaire regarding the recommended formulation and its performance. The data are analysed by the expert system founder group providing the background to further alterations and developments.

Field trials have proved that the system does provide reasonable formulations and in 1996 an updated version was available for world-wide use. Full details are given in Lai *et al.* (1996).

9.5 The Sanofi System

Personnel at the Sanofi Research Division of Philadelphia have recently developed an expert system for the formulation of hard gelatin capsules based on specific preformulation data on the active ingredient (Bateman *et al.*, 1996). The system, implemented using PFES (Chapter 3), generates one first-pass clinical capsule formulation with as many subsequent formulations as desired to accommodate an experimental design. The latter are produced as a result of the user overruling decisions made by the system.

Knowledge acquisition was by meetings between formulators with a knowledge engineer present as a consultant. Meetings were limited to two hours with minutes being taken and reviewed by all attendees. Meetings were specific to one topic defined in advance. A rapid prototyping approach was used to generate the expert system.

Knowledge in the system is structured using the strategies implemented in PFES (Chapter 3) i.e. objects and production rules. The latter are of the form:

IF (electrostatic properties of a drug are problematic)

THEN (add glidant)

UNLESS (glidant has already been added)

Tasks are scheduled dynamically. An outline of the task structure used is given in Figure 9.5.

The user is first prompted to enter specified preformulation data on the active ingredient (e.g. acid stability, molecular weight, wettability, density, particle size, hygroscopicity, melting point, solubility, etc.) and known excipient incompatibilities together with the required dose. At the initial formulation task, the capsule size is selected together with the process and milling requirements. The excipient classes are selected, some excipients being excluded and others prioritised, and their amounts determined. At the display reports task, three reports are provided, one giving the preformulation data as given, the second giving the recommended formulation including the amounts of the excipients and processing/milling requirements, and the third providing the explanation of the decisions and reasoning used by the system. On the first pass through the system the selection of the possible processing, milling and excipient options is automatic. On subsequent passes the selections are optional allowing the user to generate a number of formulations.

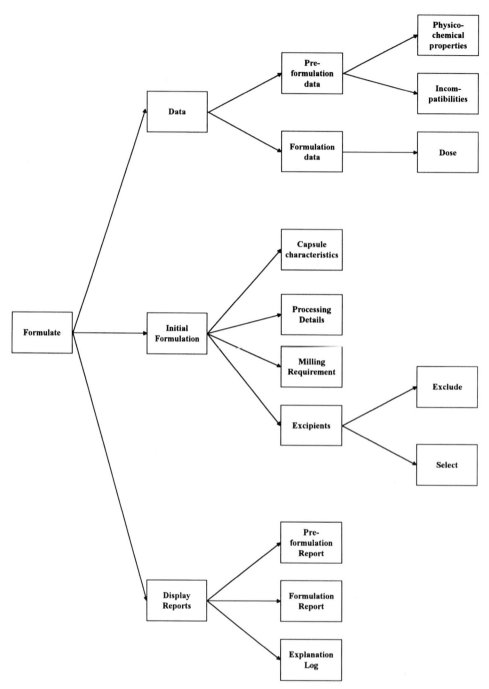

Figure 9.5 Task structure for the formulation of hard gelatin capsules as used by Bateman *et al.* (1996)

An example of a formulation for the non-steroidal anti-inflammatory drug naproxen generated by this system is given in Table 9.4. This and others were considered acceptable by experienced formulators for manufacture and initial stability evaluation.

Table 9.4 An example of a hard gelatin capsule formulation for the anti-inflammatory drug naproxen as generated by the Sanofi system (Bateman *et al.*, 1996)

Selected drug properties (inputs)

Molecular weight	230.26
Melting point (°C)	155
Solubility in water (mg ml^{-1})	0.01
Wettability	Poor
Water stability	Poor
Photostability	Poor
Susceptible to hydrolysis	No
Primary/secondary amines	No
Hygroscopicity	Class 1
Poured density (g cm^{-3})	0.366
Electrostatic problems	No
Unmilled particle size (μm)	36

Formulation

Active	Naproxen	100 mg
Diluent	Lactose (hydrous)	224 mg
Disintegrant	Microcrystalline cellulose (PH105)	60 mg
Surfactant	Sodium lauryl sulphate	4 mg
Lubricant	Talc	12 mg

Production information

Milling	Jet milling of drug
Capsule	Size 0 coloured opaque
Process	Direct blend

Explanation log

A coloured opaque capsule used because drug is unstable to light
Drug requires milling as it has a medium particle size and is insoluble
A surfactant is required because drug has poor wettability

Unfortunately Bateman *et al.* (1996) do not provide any further details on the state of the system except to imply that formulation evaluation and preformulation tasks could be accommodated with the possible development for other formulation types such as tablets, liquids and creams.

9.6 The Zeneca System

Work on expert systems within ICI (now Zeneca) Pharmaceuticals began in April 1988 with the initiation of a joint project between the Pharmaceutical and Corporate Management Services departments to investigate the use of knowledge-based techniques for the formulation of tablets. Since that time work has proceeded with the successful development of expert systems for formulating tablets, parenterals and tablet film coatings. All have been implemented using PFES from Logica UK Ltd (Chapter 3) although elements of the system developed for tablet film coatings were originally prototyped using the rule induction tool, 1st Class (Chapter 4).

Delivery of the first usable system for tablet formulation was in January 1989 (Rowe, 1993a, b). All the knowledge was acquired from two primary experts in the field of tabletting – one with extensive heuristic knowledge, the other extensive research knowledge – and structured into PFES using specialist consultancy support. Consultancy time for the initial system was of the order of 30 man days, 20 per cent of which was involved in three two-day visits to the laboratories incorporating three 90 minute interviews with the experienced formulator plus members of the research group, the demonstration of prototype systems and the validation of the previously acquired knowledge with the expert and other members of the department. Sixty per cent of the time was involved in system development and 20 per cent in writing the final report.

After commissioning and extensive demonstration to management and formulators throughout the company during 1989, the system was enhanced by the addition of a link to a database in January 1990 and the installation of a formulation optimisation routine in September 1990. A major revision was initiated in February 1991, following a significant change in formulation practice. Total consultancy time for these enhancements was of the order of 30 man days. In August 1991 the system was completed and handed over to the formulators in the UK and USA.

The completed system is shown in Figure 9.6 (Rowe, 1993a). It is divided into three stages: entry of the data, product specification and strategy; identification of the initial formulation; and formulation optimisation as a result of testing the initial formulation. The sequence is as follows:

1   The user enters all the relevant physical, chemical and mechanical properties (e.g. solubility, wettability, compatability with excipients, deformation behaviour) of the new active ingredient to be formulated into the database. The data may be numerical or symbolic; for example, for solubility in water the data can be entered as mg ml^{-1} or as the descriptors 'soluble', 'partially soluble', 'insoluble', etc. The data are obtained from a series of proprietary preformulation tests carried out on the active ingredient as received (i.e. 5 g of the drug milled to a specified particle size). These tests include excipient compatibility studies, whereby the drug is mixed with the excipient and stored under specified conditions of temperature and humidity for one week, the proportion of drug remaining being analysed by HPLC and expressed as a percentage. The deformation properties essential for the evaluation of compactability are assessed using yield pressure and strain rate sensitivity measured using a compression simulator (Rowe and Roberts, 1995).

2   The user enters the proposed dose of the active ingredient and a target tablet weight is calculated using both a formula determined from an extensive study of previously successful formulations and certain rules governing minimum weights for ease of handling and maximum weights for ease of swallowing.

3   The user selects a strategy dependent on the number of fillers (one or two).

4   The system selects the filler(s), disintegrant, binder, surfactant, glidant and lubricant and their recommended properties based on a combination of algorithms, formulae and mixture rules governing their compatibility and functionality. Tasks in this process are dynamically scheduled depending on the problem to be solved. If the system is unable to decide between two excipients which both satisfy all the embedded rules then the user is asked to select a preference.

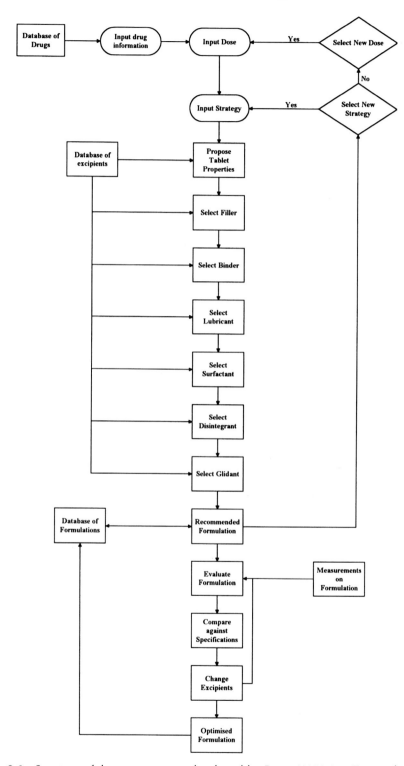

Figure 9.6 Structure of the expert system developed by Rowe (1993a) at Zeneca for the formulation of tablets

Table 9.5 Examples of tablet formulations for a model drug as generated by the Zeneca system

Drug properties (inputs)

Solubility (mg ml^{-1})	0.1
Contact angle	82°
Yield pressure (MPa)	50
Strain rate sensitivity (%)	50
+ Excipient compatibilities	

Formulation		*Quantity (mg)*	
Active	Drug A	50.0	150.0
Filler	Lactose monohydrate	166.9	–
Filler	Dicalcium phosphate dihydrate	–	165.7
Disintegrant	Crosscarmellose sodium	4.8	7.0
Binder	Polyvinylpyrrolidone	4.8	–
Binder	Hydroxypropylmethyl cellulose	–	7.0
Surfactant	Sodium lauryl sulphate	0.7	1.1
Lubricant	Magnesium stearate	2.4	3.5
Tablet weight		230.0	335.0

Predicted properties	*Formulation*	
	50 mg	*150 mg*
Tablet diameter (mm)	8.0	10.0
Yield pressure (MPa)	139	238
Strain rate sensitivity (%)	20.8	5.1

5   The recommended initial formulation is displayed including final tablet weight, recommended tablet diameter, calculated compression properties and all relevant data (Table 9.5). This is normally printed for inclusion in a laboratory notebook, file, etc. If required the data may be stored in a database for future reference, necessary if the formulation optimisation route is to be used.

6   The user enters results from testing tablets prepared using the initial formulation. These may include disintegration time, tablet strength, tablet weight variation and presence of any defects (e.g. capping, lamination, etc.). The results are compared with specifications and any problems identified are confirmed with the user. Recommendations for modifications to the formulation are then listed. This routine is fully interactive with the user who is asked to confirm or contradict/change the advice given.

7   After agreement is reached the system modifies the formulation accordingly and displays it as described above. This routine may be used as many times as required; each time the system iterates on the previously modified formulation.

Two 'Help' routines are embedded in the system, one to provide on-line help in the use of the system, the other providing an insight into the rationale behind adoption of specific rules/formulae/algorithms used. The user is able to browse the knowledge base at will but is not able to edit it without privileged access. Explanations for any recommendations made by the system can be easily accessed if required. Hypertext links are used throughout. A series of screen images from a similar system is used in Appendix 1 to illustrate the operation of a typical formulation expert system.

The system is well used and is now an integrated part of the development strategy for tablet formulation. To date it has successfully generated formulations for more than 40 active drugs. In many cases the initial formulations have been acknowledged as being on a par with those developed by expert formulators. Consequently the formulation optimisation routine is now considered redundant and very rarely used.

Following on from the successful implementation of the tablet formulation expert system, a request for the development of a similar system for parenteral formulations was made. This project was initiated in April 1992 and completed in August 1992 (Rowe *et al.*, 1995). The structure of the system is shown in Figure 9.7. It is designed for formulating a parenteral for either clinical or toxicological studies in a variety of species (dog, man, mouse, primate, rabbit or rat) by a variety of routes of administration (intravenous, intramuscular, subcutaneous, interperitoneal) supplied in either a single or multi-dose container. Knowledge was acquired from two domain experts using a series of interviews. The sequence is as follows:

1   The user enters all known data on the solubility (aqueous and non-aqueous), stability in specified solutions, compatibility, pKa and molecular properties of the active ingredient (molecular weight, Log P, etc.). As with the system for tablet formulation the data may be numerical or symbolic. All relevant properties of additives used in parenteral formulation e.g. buffers, antioxidants, chelating agents, antimicrobials and tonicity adjusters are present in the knowledge base.

2   The selection first attempts to optimise the solubility/stability of the active drug at a range of pH values using a variety of formulae and algorithms together with specific rules before selecting a buffer to achieve that pH. If problems still exist with solubility and stability then formulation variants (e.g. oil based or emulsion formulations – not implemented in the present system) are recommended.

3   The system then selects additives depending on the specification required, for example, an antimicrobial will only be added if a multi-dose container is specified or a tonicity adjuster will only be added if the solution is hypotonic. The selection strategy is generally on the basis of ranking with some specific rules.

4   The recommended formulation is displayed with all concentrations of the chosen ingredients expressed as w/v together with the calculated tonicity, proposed storage conditions and predicted shelf life (Table 9.6). Specific observations on the sensitivity of the formulation to metals, hydrolysis, light and oxygen are also included. This is normally printed for inclusion in a laboratory notebook, file, etc. If required the formulation may be stored in a database for future reference.

As with the system developed for tablet formulations, this system contains extensive 'Help' routines. No formulation optimisation routines are included although a routine to develop a placebo formulation to match the active formulation is included. The system is used to recommend parenteral formulations for a wide range of investigational drugs.

Work on expert systems in the specific domain of tablet film coating was initiated in April 1990 with the purchase of the rule induction tool, 1st Class (Chapter 4) in order to develop a system for the identification and solution of defects in film coated tablets. Although not strictly a formulation expert system, the developed

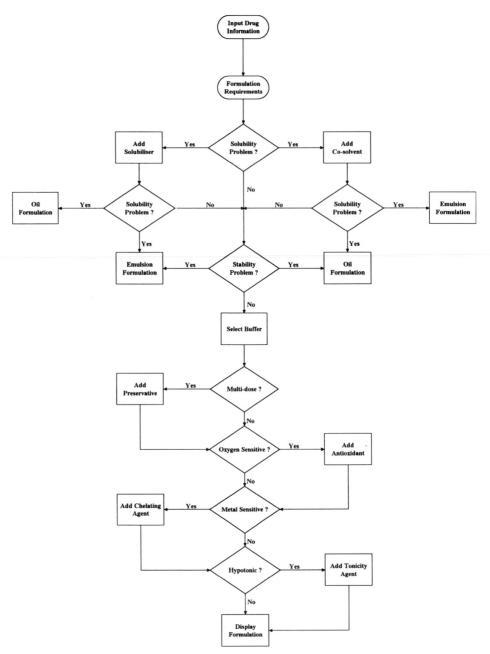

Figure 9.7 Structure of the expert system developed by Rowe *et al.* (1995) at Zeneca for the formulation of parenterals

system did contain knowledge whereby a given formulation known to cause defects could be modified to provide a solution. The completed system described by Rowe and Upjohn (1992, 1993) is a perfect illustration of fault diagnosis with a rule-based decision tree including both forward and backward chaining. Total development time was approximately one man month using both documented knowledge (Rowe, 1992) and expert assistance.

Table 9.6 An example of a formulation of an intravenous injection for clinical trials in man as generated by the Zeneca system

Drug properties (inputs)

Drug type		Acid
pKa		4.5, 3.5
Molecular weight		458.5
Solubility (mg ml^{-1})	pH 3.0	0.5
	pH 4.0	1.5
	pH 5.0	7.0
	pH 7.0	40.0
Sensitivity	Light, Metal, Oxygen	

Formulation		*Quantity (% w/v)*
Active	Drug (10 mg/ml)	1.00
Buffer	Disodium hydrogen phosphate anhydrous	0.87
Buffer	Hydrochloric acid	q.s.
Chelating agent	Disodium edetate	0.02
	Water for Injection to	100.00

Predicted solution properties

pH	7.4
Tonicity	Hypertonic (1.6)
Storage temperature (°C)	25
Atmosphere for filling	Nitrogen
Shelf life (years)	> 5

The system (Figure 9.8) is divided into three parts: identification, solution and information/references. In the first part a question and answer routine is used to ascertain the correct identification of the defect. The decision tree used for this process is shown in Figure 4.2. At this point the user is asked to confirm the decision by comparing the defect with a picture or photographs stored in the database. In the second part the user is asked to enter all relevant process conditions and formulation details regarding the best way of solving the defect. This may be a change in the process conditions as in the case of defects occurring with an already registered formulation, or a change in the formulation as in the case of defects occurring at the formulation development stage. In the third part the user is able to access data and knowledge regarding each defect. These are in the form of notes, photographs and literature references connected by hypertext links. A series of screen images from this system is used in Appendix 2 to illustrate the operation of a typical fault diagnosis expert system.

As a consequence of the successful implementation of both this system and that used to formulate tablets, it was decided in 1994 to initiate work on a new system that would recommend film coating formulations for the generated tablet formulations combined with a reformulation routine based on the film defect diagnosis system. The structure of the new system is shown in Figure 9.9; the knowledge for the system was acquired by interviewing two domain experts, one with extensive heuristic knowledge, the other with extensive research knowledge. The sequence is as follows:

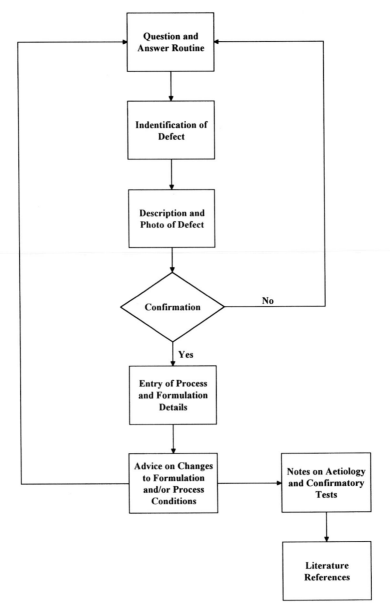

Figure 9.8 Structure of the expert system for the identification and solution of film coating defects as described by Rowe and Upjohn (1992)

1 The user enters details of the tablet formulation (e.g. dose of active ingredient and all excipients) together with all tablet properties (e.g. diameter, thickness, strength, friability, colour, shape and the presence/absence of intagliations).

2 The user enters specifications for the film coating formulation (i.e. immediate release/controlled release, enterosoluble, white or coloured).

3 The system first checks that there are not any inconsistencies between the input details and the required specification e.g. tablets with high friabilities are extremely difficult to film coat. If positive, a warning is displayed.

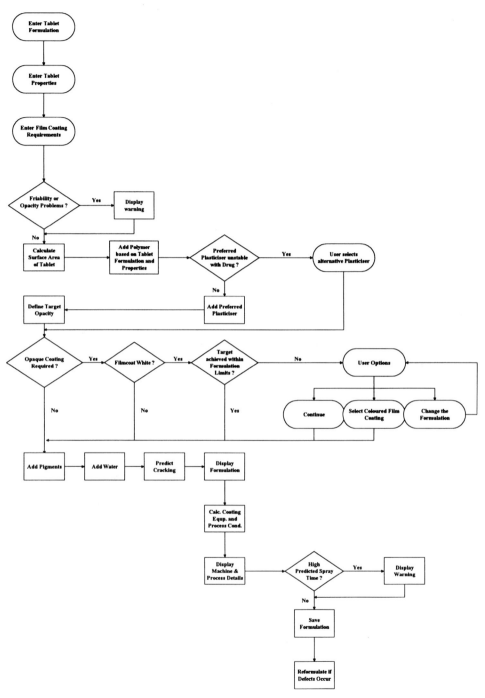

Figure 9.9 Structure of the expert system developed by Rowe *et al.* (unpublished data) at Zeneca for the formulation of tablet film coatings

Table 9.7   An example of a formulation of a white film coating for a tablet of a model drug as generated by the Zeneca system

---

Tablet properties (inputs)

Tablet core formulation	Drug A 50 mg
Punch shape	Normal concave
Weight (mg)	230
Diameter (mm)	8.0
Thickness (mm)	3.5
Surface area (cm^2)	1.49

Formulation		*mg/tab*	*mg/cm^2*
Polymer	Hydroxypropyl methylcellulose (6cps)	6.14	4.12
Plasticiser	Polyethylene glycol (PEG 400)	1.23	0.82
Pigment	Titanium dioxide (Anatase)	5.63	3.78

Predicted film properties

Thickness (µm)	45
Opacity (%)	94.9
Crack velocity (m s^{-1})	5.71

---

4   The system calculates the surface area of the tablet and selects the required polymer at the recommended level to form a film of reasonable thickness.

5   The system selects a plasticiser and checks that there are no stability/compatibility problems. If positive, the user is asked to select an alternative plasticiser.

6   The system defines the target opacity of the film coating and decides whether an opaque coating is required. The opacity is assessed by means of the contrast ratio defined as the ratio of the reflectance of the film when viewed with a black background to that viewed with a white background; the higher the value the more opaque the film (Rowe 1984a, 1984b). If positive and the specification has been set as white, the system uses specifically developed algorithms (Rowe 1995, 1996) to calculate whether the target specification can be achieved within certain predefined formulation limits of the volume concentration of titanium dioxide and film thickness. If negative, the user is provided with a series of options to continue with the predefined limits, change the limits or select a coloured film coating.

7   The system selects the pigments to achieve the target specification and determines the amount of water (the system has been developed for aqueous film coating only).

8   The system accesses a simulation program written in C to predict the cracking propensity of the film formulation (Rowe and Roberts 1992a, b; Rowe *et al.*, 1994).

9   The recommended formulation is displayed (Table 9.7), including predicted film thickness, opacity and cracking propensity. Standard machine settings and process details are also displayed with warnings if the total spray time is judged to be excessive. This is normally printed for inclusion in a laboratory notebook or file. If required and in particular if reformulation is likely to be necessary the data may be stored in a database for future reference.

10 If reformulation is necessary due to the presence of defects after coating, then the system uses a modified form of the defect diagnosis system to recommend changes in the formulation and/or process conditions.

The system has proved successful in initial trials especially in the formulation of opaque films for drugs that are either unstable to light or are coloured, producing mottled tablets. The calculations concerning the achievement of the target opacity within predefined limits have enabled formulators to make informed decisions regarding the use of white or coloured film coatings. The system is now an integral part of the development strategy for film coated tablets and has a common database with the tablet formulation system.

9.7 Conclusion

It can be seen that expert systems have now been developed by a number of pharmaceutical companies and academic institutes covering all the most common formulation types. Only those that have been mentioned in the open literature have been discussed although it is generally known that other systems have been developed by SmithKline Beecham, Wellcome (now Glaxo Wellcome), Eli Lilly and Pfizer. There are possibly many more, but reticence regarding publication abounds and it is difficult to estimate exactly the number developed. The impact and benefits as well as the issues surrounding their implementation will be discussed in Chapters 11 and 12 respectively.

References

BATEMAN, S.D., VERLIN, J., RUSSO, M., GUILLOT, M. and LAUGHLIN, S.M., 1996, The development and validation of a capsule formulation knowledge-based system, *Pharm. Technol.*, **20** (3), 174–184.

BRADSHAW, D., 1989, The computer learns from the experts, *Financial Times*, London, 27 April.

CARR, R., 1965, Evaluating flow properties of solids, *Chem. Engineer*, **18**, 163–168.

FRANK, J., RUPPRECHT, B. and SCHMELMER, V., 1997, Knowledge-based assistance for the development of drugs, *IEEE Expert*, **12** (1), 40–48.

LAI, S., PODCZECK, F., NEWTON, J.M. and DAUMESNIL, R., 1995, An expert system for the development of powder filled hard gelatin capsule formulations, *Pharm. Res.*, **12** (9), S150.

LAI, S., PODCZECK, F., NEWTON, J.M. and DAUMESNIL, R., 1996, An expert system to aid the development of capsule formulations, *Pharm. Tech. Eur.*, **8** (9), 60–68.

LUDDE, K.H. and KAWAKITA, K., 1966, Die pulverkompression, *Pharmazie*, **21**, 393–403.

RAMANI, K.V., PATEL, M.R. and PATEL, S.K., 1992, An expert system for drug preformulation in a pharmaceutical company, *Interfaces*, **22** (2), 101–108.

ROWE, R.C., 1984a, The opacity of tablet film coatings, *J. Pharm. Pharmac.*, **36**, 569–572.

ROWE, R.C., 1984b, Quantitative opacity measurements on tablet film coatings containing titanium dioxide, *Int. J. Pharm.*, **22**, 17–23.

ROWE, R.C., 1992, Defects in film coated tablets – aetiology and solution, in GANDERTON, D. and JONES, T. (eds), *Advances in Pharmaceutical Sciences*, Vol. 6, pp. 65–100, London: Academic Press.

ROWE, R.C., 1993a, An expert system for the formulation of pharmaceutical tablets, *Manufacturing Intelligence*, **14**, 13–15.

ROWE, R.C., 1993b, Expert systems in solid dosage development, *Pharm. Ind.*, **55**, 1040–1045.

ROWE, R.C., 1995, Knowledge representation in the prediction of the opacity of tablet film coatings containing titanium dioxide, *Eur. J. Pharm. Biopharm.*, **41**, 215–218.

ROWE, R.C., 1996, Predicting film thickness on film coated tablets, *Int. J. Pharm.*, **133**, 253–256.

ROWE, R.C. and ROBERTS, R.J., 1992a, Simulation of crack propagation in tablet film coatings containing pigments, *Int. J. Pharm.*, **78**, 49–57.

ROWE, R.J. and ROBERTS, R.J., 1992b, The effect of some formulation variables on crack propagation in pigmented tablet film coatings using computer simulation, *Int. J. Pharm.*, **86**, 49–58.

ROWE, R.C. and ROBERTS, R.J., 1995, The mechanical properties of powders, in GANDERTON, D., JONES, T. and McGINITY, J. (eds), *Advances in Pharmaceutical Sciences*, Vol. 7, pp. 1–62, London: Academic Press.

ROWE, R.C. and UPJOHN, N.G., 1992, An expert system for identifying and solving defects on film-coated tablets, *Manufacturing Intelligence*, **12**, 12–13.

ROWE, R.C. and UPJOHN, N.G., 1993, An expert system for the identification and solution of film coating defects, *Pharm. Tech. Int.*, **5** (3), 34–38.

ROWE, R.C., ROWE, M.D. and ROBERTS, R.J., 1994, Formulating film coatings with the aid of computer simulations, *Pharm. Technol.*, **18** (10), 132–139.

ROWE, R.C., WAKERLY, M.G., ROBERTS, R.J., GRUNDY, R.U. and UPJOHN, N.G., 1995, Expert system for parenteral development, *PDA. J. Pharm. Sci. Technol.*, **49**, 257–261.

STRICKER, H., HAUX, R., WETTER, T., MANN, G., OBERHAMMER, L., FLISTER, J., FUCHS, S. and SCHMELMER, V., 1991, Das Galenische Entwicklungs – System Heidelberg, *Pharm. Ind.*, **53**, 571–578.

STRICKER, H., FUCHS, S., HAUX, R., ROSSLER, R., RUPPRECHT, B., SCHMELMER, V. and WIEGEL, S., 1994, Das Galenische Entwicklungs – System Heidelberg – Systematische Rezepturentwicklung, *Pharm. Ind.*, **56**, 641–647.

WALKO, J.Z., 1989, Turning Dalton's theory into practice, *Innovation*, pp. 18, 24, London: ICI Europa Ltd.

WELLS, J., 1988, *Pharmaceutical Preformulation – The Physicochemical Properties of Drug Substances*, Chichester: Ellis Horwood.

10

Applications of Neural Networks and Genetic Algorithms

10.1 Introduction

The properties of a formulation are determined not only by the ratios in which the ingredients are combined but also by the processing conditions. Although relationships between ingredient levels, processing conditions and product performance may be known anecdotally, rarely can they be quantified. Neural networks and genetic algorithms offer a rapid and easy way of modelling and optimising formulations in multidimensional space.

Such systems are now in use in many areas of product formulation by many companies (Table 10.1). Unfortunately many are reticent about revealing information on their experience and hence only a limited number of case studies are in the open literature – for adhesives, paints and coatings and pharmaceutical tablets.

10.2 Adhesives

An adhesive can be defined as a material or composition capable of holding together solid materials (adherends) by means of a surface attachment. When high strength materials (e.g. metals) are used as the adherends and the bonded joint is capable of bearing loads of considerable magnitude the adhesive is known as a structural adhesive. These are the strongest forms of adhesives and are designed to bear loads permanently. They are generally resin compositions containing a variety of additives e.g. promoters, curing aids, elastomeric modifers, activators, antioxidants and wetting agents and can be applied as liquids, pastes or even solids. For any application the adhesive must meet a variety of potentially conflicting requirements such as bond strength, thermal stability, resistance to corrosion, water, and light, etc., ability to adhere to dirty or oily surfaces, ease of application and cost. Formulating an optimised adhesive is thus a challenging task.

In an attempt to provide customers with an adhesive that would not only form thermally stable bonds to a number of different substrates but also meet certain manufacturing constraints, personnel at the Lord Corporation (Chemical Products

Table 10.1 Some representative applications and users of neural networks and genetic algorithms (data courtesy of AI Ware Inc.) (all companies from USA unless stated)

Industry	Application	Company
Adhesives	Specialty adhesives	Avery International
		H.B. Fuller Co.
		Lord Corporation
		Morton International
Biotechnology	Cell culture media	Hyclone Laboratories
Composites	Friction materials	Advanced Ceramics
	Thermoset moulding	Allied Signal
	compounds	Ciba Composites (UK)
	Ceramics	Premix
Food	Confectionary	Kraft General Foods
	Flavours/fragrances	Quest International (Holland)
		Warner Lambert
Paints and coatings	Paints	Courtaulds (UK)
	Coatings	EI DuPont De Nemours
	Inks	ICI (UK)
		The Glidden Paint Company
		Xerox Corporation
Pharmaceutical/medical	Pharmaceuticals	Eli Lilly and Company
	Diagnostics	Miles Laboratories
		Zeneca Pharmaceuticals (UK)
Plastics	Specialty polymers	Air Products and Chemicals
	Resins	BASF Corporation
	Fibres	BF Goodrich
		Dow Corning SA (Holland)
		Dow Chemical
		DSM Resins (Holland)
		Hoechst Celanese
		Monsanto Company
Rubber	Tyres	Columbian Chemicals
	Carbon black	Cooper Tyre Company
		Goodyear Tyre and Rubber Co
Specialty chemicals	Household chemicals	Albright and Wilson (UK)
	Industrial chemicals	Asahi Chemical (Japan)
	Water treatment chemicals	Betz Laboratories
		Daicel Chemical (Japan)
		Hitachi Chemical (Japan)
		Procter and Gamble
		Mitsubishi Chemical America
		Reckitt and Coleman (UK)
		SC Johnson Wax
		Zeneca Specialties (UK)

Division) USA have used CAD/Chem from AI Ware Inc. (Chapter 6) to model and optimise a new product (Gill and Shutt, 1992; VerDuin, 1994). It was already known that a specific additive, a promoter, at different concentrations could produce thermally stable bonds to different substrates. However, the promoter was known to be a mixture of various reaction products, the distribution of which depended on the manufacturing process and which, although they did promote adhesion when included in small amounts, in larger concentrations were detrimental.

Developing a statistical model relating the product formulation and resulting properties was not an option since there was no way to control all of the components in the formulation independently (the amounts of the various reaction products in the promoter were fixed in relation to each other by the manufacturing process). Hence a neural network approach was chosen. The network was trained using data from 38 formulations with seven different lots of the promoter at varying concentration, each lot having been previously analysed to determine its composition. Other than that the network had a feed forward three layer (a single hidden layer) architecture no further details are available. The model once generated was optimised with constraints on the ratios of various of the components of the promoter at levels which could be produced by the current manufacturing process. Laboratory evaluation of the optimum formulation confirmed its properties as the best product.

An unconstrained search was also introduced to predict the optimum distribution of the components in the promoter which might provide an even better level of performance. This was used by the company to investigate whether or not it was cost effective to change the manufacturing process for the promoter in order to produce a better adhesive.

The project was regarded as being very successful since, by using the neural network and genetic algorithm approach, a formulation was identified within days as compared with the one year already expended. In addition, the additional information from the unconstrained search provided targets for future research and development into the process of manufacturing the promoter (Gill and Shutt, 1992).

10.3 Paints and Coatings

Paints and coatings are ubiquitous. They are used for decorative, protective and functional treatments of a wide range of surfaces. Architectural coatings and household paints are used mainly for decoration, while marine coatings (e.g. for undersea pipelines) are generally used for protective purposes. Others such as exterior automobile coatings fulfil both decorative and protective functions. Many specialised coatings are for specific functions e.g. the control of fouling on keels of ships, the protection of food and beverages in cans, and the magnetic coatings on videotapes. All coatings are formulated from four basic components: one or more resins or binders (e.g. alkyds, polyesters, acrylic resins, epoxy resins, urethanes, etc.); pigments and extenders (e.g. titanium dioxide, coloured pigments, calcium carbonate, and clays); solvents (e.g. ketones, esters, alcohols and water) not used for powder coatings; and frequently special additives (e.g. catalysts, crosslinkers, thickeners, biocides, fungicides, dispersants, surfactants, defoamers, light stabilisers, antioxidants, ultraviolet absorbers, etc.). Coatings are formulated for mechanical properties (e.g. hardness, elasticity); adhesion to substrates; resistance to wear, acid, sunlight, various chemicals and solvents, ease of application, and cost. Statistical formulation methods and considerable experimentation are often needed to determine how a change in the formulation will change the product properties. Recently neural networks have been applied to two problems.

In the first, a relatively simple acid resistance study performed by Glidden Research Centre, USA (Gill and Shutt, 1992; VerDuin, 1994), seven formulation

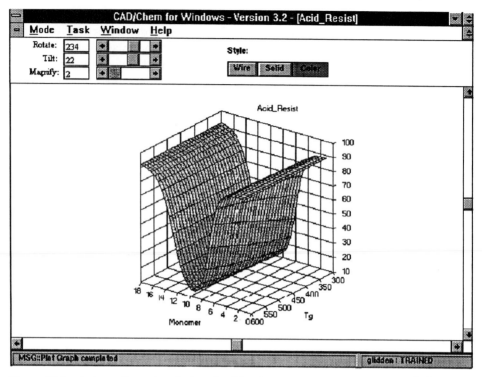

Figure 10.1 A three-dimensional plot of acid resistance, monomer content and glass transition temperature for a paint formulation showing two optima (by permission AI Ware Inc.)

variables (including crosslinker level and monomer content) and three perform-ance variables (two being the acid resistance measured by two different methods) were evaluated using 24 experiments in an experimental design.

Using CAD/Chem, Gill and Shutt (1992) were able to model the system using a single layer neural network. Once desirability functions were set so as to maximise the value of the first test to measure acid resistance and minimise the value of the second test, an unconstrained optimisation using the genetic algorithm was under-taken. Unexpectedly, the search found an optimum outside the experimentally mapped space where the glass transition temperature and crosslinker levels were below the range specified by the formulator in setting up the experimental design. A further optimisation, this time constrained to restrict the levels of the glass transition temperature and crosslinker levels to the range originally specified by the formulator, found a different optimum. This formulation had a glass transition temperature and crosslinker levels in the middle of their specified range but the level of monomer had changed from 22 per cent to 0.9 per cent.

A close scrutiny of these apparently anomalous results revealed that a plot of the first acid resistance test against monomer level and glass transition temperature had a response surface with two peaks of nearly equal magnitude (Figure 10.1). Constraining the search space to just the experimentally explored region excluded the global optimum and only included the lower local optimum. The data were shown to the formulator who confirmed that there had been past evidence that both high and low levels of monomer sometimes gave good properties. He also indicated that the only reason the glass transition temperature and crosslinker levels had been specified was because prior experience had shown them to be the best. On the basis of this finding a new programme of work was undertaken to formulate at lower glass transition temperature and crosslinker levels in order to reduce the level of the expensive monomer while still retaining high performance in respect of acid resistance. The process resulted in significant cost savings.

In a second application, Zupan and Gasteiger (1993) reported work carried out by personnel at the National Institute of Chemistry in Ljubljana, Slovenia for a chemical factory producing paints. They found that for the product investigated there were three highly significant and non-correlated variables, i.e. the polymer concentration, catalyst concentration and temperature used to heat the product, with six properties to be controlled i.e. paint hardness, elasticity, adhesion, resistance to methyl-isobutyl ketone, stroke resistance and contra-stroke resistance. An experimental design was selected involving the preparation of 27 samples of paint. All properties were assessed on a quality scale in which 1.0 represented superior quality and 0.0 represented extremely poor or unmeasurable quality.

A neural network having three input neurons, 20 hidden neurons in the hidden layer and six output neurons was trained with the data for about 10 000 epochs. After training, two-dimensional maps (each at a constant value of the third parameter) were produced for evaluation. No further details regarding the use of the data in the optimisation of a formulation were given.

10.4 Pharmaceuticals

To date all applications in this domain have been in the area of tablets covering both immediate release and controlled release formulations.

The first work to be carried out was by Hussain and coworkers at the University of Cincinnati on modelling the *in-vitro* release rate characteristics of a variety of drugs from matrices prepared from hydrophilic polymers. In the first study (Hussain *et al.*, 1991) the release of the antihistamine drug chlorpheniramine maleate (25% w/w) from matrices of sodium carboxymethylcellulose, hydroxypropyl methylcellulose, hydroxypropyl cellulose and hydroxyethyl cellulose singly and as blends was modelled using a generic neural network simulator. Four formulation variables corresponding to combinations of the hydrophilic polymers and two response variables (the release exponential and the dissolution half-time) constituted the input and output layers of the network. The optimum number of neurons in the single hidden layer was selected by training the network with a single hidden layer containing 4, 6, 8, 10, 12 and 14 neurons and evaluating the residual sum of the squared error. The network with eight hidden neurons was found to be the best. The network was trained with 15 formulations using a learning rate of 0.25 and a momentum factor of 0.9 with all input and output data scaled within the 0.1–0.9 range to conform to the software format. A test set of eight formulations was used to validate the model. Residuals (i.e. experimental minus predicted result) for both the release exponential and dissolution half-time showed that the neural network was able to predict these response values more precisely than response methodology.

In a follow-up study Hussain *et al.* (1992) used literature data for 28 drugs dispersed in matrices of hydroxypropyl methylcellulose of varying molecular weight (40 formulations in total). A three layer feed-forward network containing 13 input neurons corresponding *inter alia* to viscosity of polymer, molecular weight of drug, solubility of drug, ionic character of drug, salt type, tablet diameter, weight, drug/ polymer ratio), three hidden neurons and two output neurons corresponding to the release exponential, and dissolution half-life was constructed using Neural Ware Professional from Neural Ware Inc. and trained with 29 formulations for 2900 iterations. A comparison of predictions for the 11 test formulations showed good correlation for the dissolution half-time but for the release exponential one predic- tion had a high unexplained residual error.

In a third study Hussain *et al.* (1994) used the same software package to train a network consisting of three layers, with six input neurons (drug molecular weight, intrinsic dissolution rate, pKa, salt type, drug/polymer ratio and polymer hydration rate), six hidden neurons and four output neurons (percentage drug released at 1, 3, 6 and 12 hours). The selection of six hidden neurons was based on experimenta- tion to minimise the root mean square error. Formulations comprising binary mixes of sodium salts of the anti-inflammatory drugs diclofenac, naproxen and salicylic acid, the hydrochloride salts of the antihistamine drug diphenhydramine, the sym- pathomimetic agent phenylpropanolamine, the cholinesterase inhibitor tetrahydro- aminoacridine, the beta-adrenergic blocking agent propranolol, the stimulants caffeine and theophylline, the analgesic drug paracetamol (acetaminophen) and the cardiac depressant quinidine sulphate together with hydroxypropyl cellulose, characterised by three hydration times in three drug/polymer ratios, were compressed using a single punch machine with standard biconcave tooling (11 mm diameter) to a weight of 350 mg and a strength 10–15 Kp. *In-vitro* release rate profiles were measured in deionised water at 37°C. The entire data set was used to train the network and the trained network was validated by evaluating its ability to predict the release pro- file using a 'one-out' method i.e. removing a single formulation from the training set, retraining the network and then predicting the release profile of the removed formulation.

While the network was able to predict, with acceptable accuracy, the release profiles of all the sodium salts, caffeine, theophylline, paracetamol and the hydro- chloride salts with the exception of that of phenylpropanolamine, it was unable to predict those for quinidine sulphate. When predictions outside its domain were attempted the performance was poor.

No attempt was made by the authors to optimise the formulations using genetic algorithms or any other procedure but the results have led them to propose the concept of computer aided formulation design based on neural networks (Hussain *et al.*, 1994).

In a study to examine the effects of lubricant type, duration of mixing and tab- let compression pressure on drug release rates, Turkoglu and coworkers from the University of Marmara, Istanbul, Turkey and the University of Cincinnati used both neural networks and statistics for data analysis (Turkoglu *et al.*, 1995). The tablets were composed of 25 mg of the diuretic drug hydrochlorothiazide, 272 mg of microcrystalline cellulose as diluent and 3 mg of the lubricant magnesium stearate, glyceryl behenate and a blend of equal parts talc and magnesium stearate. All materials were mixed in a V-shaped blender for three different mixing times (10, 40 and 160 minutes) and directly compressed at three different compression pres- sures (31, 63 and 94 MPa) using 9 mm shallow concave punches. Drug release in 0.1N HCl at 37°C was measured at two time points (30 and 60 minutes) and tablet

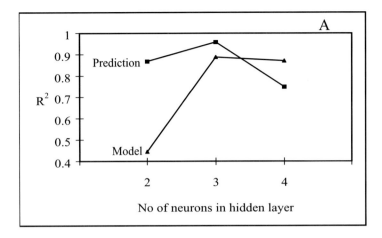

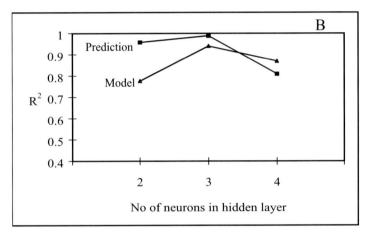

Figure 10.2 Effect of number of neurons in the hidden layer (X) on R^2 values for the 3–X–3 (A) and the 3–X–2 (B) networks for both the model and the prediction of drug release at 60 minutes (data from Turkoglu *et al.*, 1995)

strength measured for tablets produced at the three compression pressures. A total of 27 experiments were run; 22 were used for training the neural network, the remainder were used for testing.

Three layer neural networks, each with inputs of lubricant type, mixing time and compression pressure and a single hidden layer with two, three and four neurons and an output layer of either three neurons (drug release at two time points and tablet strength) or two neurons (drug release at two time points) were constructed using DANA (Design Advisor/Neural Analyser) from Neural Ware Inc. For both networks, those containing three hidden neurons gave the best models (Figure 10.2).

The networks produced were used to produce three-dimensional plots of mixing time, compression pressure and crushing strength, or drug release, mixing time and compression pressure in an attempt to optimise the formulation to maximise tablet strength or to select the best lubricant types. Although trends were observed no optimal formulations were given. The output was comparable to that using multiple regression analysis.

In a more extensive evaluation of neural networks to model tablet formulations, Kesavan and Peck (1995) from Procter and Gamble Pharmaceuticals and Purdue University used a formulation comprising 40% w/w of the stimulant drug anhydrous caffeine, 44.5–47.5% w/w of either dicalcium phosphate dihydrate or lactose mono-hydrate as diluents and 2.0–5.0% w/w of polyvinyl pyrrolidone as a binder. Granules were prepared on two types of granulating equipment – a fluidised bed and a high shear mixer-granulator with the binder being added either as an aqueous solution or a dry powder. The geometric mean size, flow value, bulk and tapped densities of the dry granules were measured. The dry granules were blended together with 10% w/w of corn starch as a disintegrant and 0.5% w/w of magnesium stearate as a lubricant and compressed at 128 MPa, producing tablets which were tested for strength, friability, thickness and disintegration time. Thirty-two experiments were run; 24 were used to train the network and the remainder were used for testing the network.

Two networks were developed, one comprising five inputs (diluent type, diluent level, binder level, granulation equipment and binder addition wet or dry), the other comprising nine inputs (the five above plus granule size, flow, bulk and tapped densities). Both networks had a single hidden layer of five neurons and an output layer of four neurons (tablet strength, friability, thickness and disintegration time). Both were constructed using generic software with correlations between observed and predicted results generally better than those seen with regression analysis.

These same data have been reanalysed by Colbourn and Rowe (1996) using CAD/Chem from AI Ware Inc. (Chapter 6). Not only were the authors able to show that the models generated by the software were comparable with those developed by Kesavan and Peck (1995) but also that networks with four and six neuron hidden layer architectures gave comparable results.

From the data a five neuron single hidden layer neural network was used to generate a model relating the input formulation and processing conditions to the final tablet properties. For this model four different optimisations were investigated by varying the weights which describe the relative importance of the four tablet properties (Table 10.2). Constraints were applied to restrict the levels of both the diluent and binder concentrations to those tested and to include the requirement that the diluent type, granulation equipment and binder addition (wet or dry) had to be integral values (1 or 2). This was to reflect the fact that these parameters switched between two different values and that a non-integral value would be mean-ingless. The optimisations were carried out to maximise tablet strength, minimum tablet friability and disintegration time and restrict tablet thickness between 2.8 and 3.4 mm.

In all cases (Table 10.2) lactose was the preferred diluent and the binder concentration was in the lower half of the design range consistent with decreasing friability and disintegration time. Little change was seen with the tablet strength; the only way in which a high strength could be obtained was at the expense of the other variables, particularly the disintegration time. Interestingly, when strength was assigned a property weight of 10 and disintegration time a weight of 5, the binder addition changed from wet to dry (Table 10.2).

In the most recent application of neural networks in the formulation of tab-lets, personnel from the pharmaceutical company KRKA d.d. and the University of Ljubljana, Slovenia, have used the technique to optimise release of the anti-

Table 10.2 Input weights (i.e. relative importance) and results of four optimisation runs for a tablet formulation (Colbourn and Rowe, 1996)

Optimisation run no.	1	2	3	4
		Input weights		
Tablet strength	9	9	5	10
Tablet friability	9	5	2	2
Tablet thickness	5	5	2	2
Disintegration time	10	10	10	10
Results				
Diluent type	←———————— Lactose ————————→			
Diluent conc. (% w/w)	49.98	49.99	50.0	49.59
PVP (% w/w)	3.55	3.29	2.15	3.03
Binder addition	Wet	Wet	Wet	Dry
Equipment	←———————— Fluidised bed ————————→			
Predictions				
Tablet strength (kp)	9.96	9.96	9.96	12.11
Tablet friability (%)	0.57	0.73	0.84	0.03
Tablet thickness (mm)	3.29	3.29	3.29	2.86
Disintegration time (s)	250	210	197	900

inflammatory drug diclofenac sodium from sustained release tablets (Zupancic Bozic *et al.*, 1997). The formulation comprised drug, sucrose, cetyl alcohol (19.4–27.4%), polyvinyl pyrrolidone (0.2–7.0%), magnesium stearate (0.2–1.5%) and colloidal silica. Release of the drug into phosphate buffer at pH 6.8 was measured over a period of six hours, samples being taken at 19 time points. A multilayer perceptron with an input layer of four neurons representing the amounts of cetyl alcohol, polyvinyl pyrrolidone, magnesium stearate and time, an output layer of one neuron representing the amount of drug released at the stated time point and a hidden layer of 12 neurons was trained for 10^5 epochs using back-propagation. The training time using bespoke software was ten hours.

The model was used both for consultation and optimisation using two- and three-dimensional response surface analysis. Non-linear relationships were found offering the possibility of producing several formulations with the same release rate.

10.5 Conclusion

The applications clearly show the range and complexity of the formulations to which neural networks and/or genetic algorithms can be directed. Where models generated using neural networks have been compared with those generated using statistical techniques, the results were either equivalent or better. The latter was specifically valid where the applications were multi-dimensional in nature and where variables exhibited interdependencies (e.g. in the formulation used by Kesavan and Peck, 1995). When genetic algorithms were used for optimisation, constraints and preferences could be easily accommodated allowing any number of optimised formulations to be developed. Benefits and impacts will be discussed in Chapter 11.

References

COLBOURN, E.A. and ROWE, R.C., 1996, Modelling and optimisation of a tablet formulation using neural networks and genetic algorithms, *Pharm. Tech. Eur.*, **8** (9), 46–55.

GILL, T. and SHUTT, J., 1992, Optimising product formulations using neural networks, *Scientific Computing and Automation*, **5** (9), 19–26.

HUSSAIN, A.S., YU, X. and JOHNSON, R.D., 1991, Application of neural computing in pharmaceutical product development, *Pharm. Res.*, **8**, 1248–1252.

HUSSAIN, A.S., JOHNSON, R.D. and SHIVANAND, P., 1992, Artificial neural network based system for predicting the in-vitro drug release from hydroxypropyl methylcellulose matrix tablets, *Proc. 11th Pharm. Tech. Conf.*, **2**, 74–76.

HUSSAIN, A.S., SHIVANAND, P. and JOHNSON, R.D., 1994, Application of neural computing in pharmaceutical product development: computer aided formulation design, *Drug Dev. Ind. Pharm.*, **20**, 1739–1752.

KESAVAN, J.G. and PECK, G.E., 1995, Pharmaceutical formulation using neural networks, *Proc. 14th Pharm. Tech. Conf.*, **2**, 413–431.

TURKOGLU, M., OZARSLAN, R. and SAKR, A., 1995, Artificial neural network analysis of a direct compression tabletting study, *Eur. J. Pharm. Biopharm.*, **41**, 315–322.

VERDUIN, W.H., 1994, Knowledge-based systems for formulation optimisation, *Tappi*, **77**, 100–104.

ZUPAN, J. and GASTEIGER, J., 1993, *Neural networks for chemists – an introduction*, pp. 221–227, Weinheim: VCH.

ZUPANCIC BOZIC, D., VRECER, F. and KOZJEK, F., 1997, Optimisation of diclofenac sodium dissolution from sustained release formulations using an artificial neural network, *Eur. J. Pharm. Sci.*, **5**, 163–169.

11

Benefits and Impact of Intelligent Software

11.1 Introduction

There is still much uncertainty about the benefits of introducing intelligent software generally, let alone specifically, in the domain of product formulation although there is a great deal of interest in developments of the technology and applications.

The situation does not appear to have changed much since 1989 when a large survey specifically on expert systems applications involving nearly 450 responses from a wide variety of organisations from all sectors of business in the UK revealed that 52 per cent of the organisations had only a watching brief and that only 11 per cent had operational systems (Figure 11.1). Since this result was expected to be biased in favour of interested organisations it was concluded that there was a high level of anxiety (Dewar, 1989).

Since relatively high investments of time and resources are often needed to develop systems it is imperative that benefits, if any, be identified and assessed objectively. From an understanding of these benefits and the costs involved in developing the application a cost/benefit analysis can be carried out.

Benefits from intelligent software can be broadly divided into two groups:

1 Potential benefits – those predicted from a knowledge of the underlying technology (i.e. artificial intelligence). In many cases these are extrapolated by enthusiasts to produce exaggerated claims for a business impact.

2 Proven or identifiable benefits – those observed by analysing the application and its use in the real world. Often these are very similar to the potential benefits but in many cases more are highlighted. These may be subdivided into two further categories:

   - measurable benefits, the value of which can be measured or estimated in quantitative, often economic terms;
   - non-measurable benefits (often referred to as intangibles), the economic value of which cannot be measured but only appreciated in qualitative terms.

In this chapter the benefits of both expert systems and neural networks/genetic algorithms are assessed.

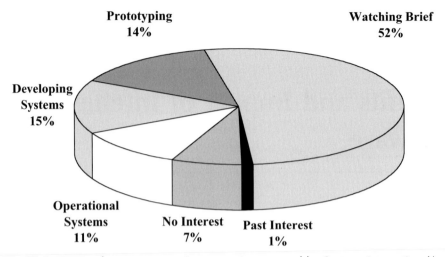

Prototyping
14%

Watching Brief
52%

Developing
Systems
15%

Operational
Systems
11%

No Interest
7%

Past Interest
1%

Figure 11.1 Status of expert systems in companies surveyed by Systems International/es (Connect) as reported by Dewar (1989)

11.2 Expert Systems

Potential benefits of expert systems arise from the predicted advantages of artificial intelligence (Chapter 1) as follows:

- Permanence i.e. knowledge in an expert system is permanent, non-perishable and not affected by staff turnover. This benefit has been extrapolated to that of fewer skilled staff.
- Ease of duplication and dissemination i.e. knowledge in an expert system can be easily transferred across international borders in a form accessible to all. This benefit has been extrapolated to a reduced skill level.
- Consistency and reliability i.e. expert systems use all available, relevant information and do not overlook potential solutions. This benefit has been extrapolated to better quality of work.
- Ease of documentation i.e. decisions made in expert systems can be easily documented by tracing all the activities of the system. This benefit has been extrapolated to a training aid for novices.
- Rapid response i.e. computers can perform tasks at ever increasing speeds. This benefit has been extrapolated to increased output.
- Lower expense i.e. computer hardware is becoming less expensive. This benefit has been extrapolated to reduced costs.

Hence, if the exaggerated claims are to be believed, expert systems should result in the wider availability of scarce knowledge, increased output, fewer skilled staff, lower skill levels, increased quality but at reduced costs. Of course, the wider availability of scarce knowledge is only a benefit if the knowledge is valuable and its limited availability is limiting the performance of the company. However, these potential benefits and exaggerated claims have been so well disseminated that they have become generally accepted as fact by potential users. For instance, in one survey by Tinsley (1992), among a sample of small/medium UK companies in manufacturing and process industries, none of which were actively using expert

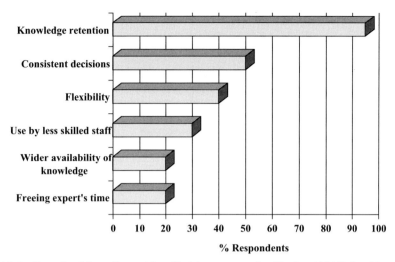

Figure 11.2   Perceived benefits as identified in a survey by Tinsley (1992) for 20 small/ medium companies in the UK, none of which were using expert systems

systems although some 60 per cent had a general awareness of the technology, the perceived benefits were as shown in Figure 11.2. The benefit most commonly associated with expert systems was their use as a way of retaining specialised knowledge. Others identified were:

- improvement in the quality of work;
- flexibility of expert systems;
- expert tasks can be undertaken by less skilled staff;
- specialist knowledge can be made more widely available in the organisation;
- specialist staff are freed from routine work.

However, in a much larger survey in 1989 by Systems International/es (Connect) involving nearly 450 responses from a wide variety of organisations and types of users (Dewar, 1989), the identified benefits included many more factors considered key to the applications (Figure 11.3). The data were also analysed by a number of segments, the two most relevant being the status of the system (idea through to operational system) and the intended user (to support a lay person or knowledgeable user) (Figures 11.4 and 11.5). The former was important since it revealed the changing attitude to benefits as the system evolved. It was significant that 57 per cent of the systems were intended to be used by a knowledgeable user and the benefits reflected this fact.

Overall the most important benefits were those concerned with the accuracy of the decision making and improved problem solving, quality/accuracy of work. This pattern was found to be consistent over all segments except in the case of knowledgeable users where accuracy of work was more important and in the case where human operators were being replaced where improved problem solving was not important.

The less important benefits were those concerned with the reduction in staff numbers or using less skilled staff. This reflected the 57 per cent of systems intended for knowledgeable users where cost savings were not important if there were

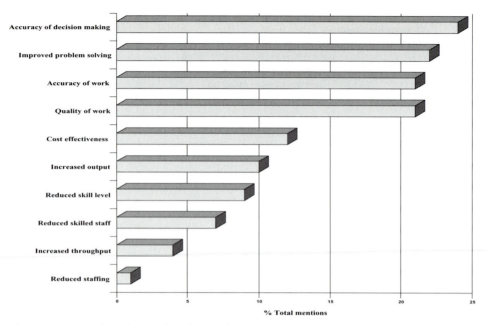

Figure 11.3 Key benefits as identified in the Systems International/es (Connect) survey of expert systems applications as reported by Dewar (1989)

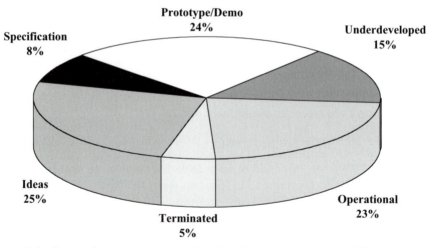

Figure 11.4 Status of expert systems applications in companies surveyed by Systems International/es (Connect) as reported by Dewar (1989)

other intangible benefits. However, for other users of systems i.e. those included to advise a lay person, reduced skill level was considered more important. Cost effectiveness was found to vary with stage of development with a greater focus on this benefit as development proceeded.

When benefits were analysed for systems at the idea stage, the same trends were revealed. It was concluded that developers did not necessarily set out to achieve cost savings but to improve how the tasks were performed. Very few applications at the ideas stage were identified as being intended to replace a human but the proportion did increase through the development stage (Dewar, 1989).

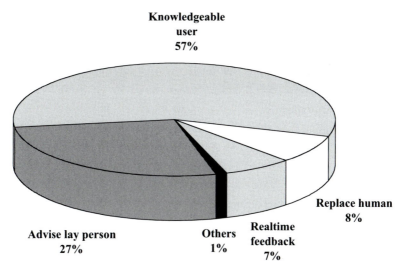

Figure 11.5 Intended users of expert systems applications in companies surveyed by Systems International/es (Connect) as reported by Dewar (1989)

In another survey, this time involving 12 fully operational systems in manufacturing, engineering, medical and finance, Shaw (1990) divided the benefits into those relative to infrastructure, people, efficiency/productivity and external competitiveness (Figure 11.6). No attempt was made to analyse the findings with respect to the type of system implemented. If this had been done the low value ascribed to equipment utilisation would have been much higher since only 42 per cent of the systems surveyed dealt with equipment usage. Nine out of 12 companies reported a reduced capital/overhead cost with 10 of the 12 reporting better management control, better image/client service, more time to undertake new activities or develop new products and improved competitiveness.

It is interesting to note that 11 of the 12 provided details of overall business impact in directly quantifiable terms. Two reported a payback in under six months, four between six and 12 months, two between one and two years and three between two and four years.

Benefits not explicitly reported in any of the surveys but mentioned by Tinsley (1992) as a result of his discussions with companies included:

- Savings through reduced error and wastage.
- Better utilisation of materials.
- An opportunity to re-examine activities.

The last benefit arose out of the process of identifying and developing a system for the activity. Some companies found that it was the first time they had studied the activity in detail.

Thomas (1991) has attempted to capture the overall impact of expert system technology within an organisation in terms of the quality, availability and consistency of expertise as shown in Figure 11.7. He suggests that managers should, as the diagram suggests, move the focus of attention from the technology itself to its business impact. Expert systems should enable organisations to begin to manage expertise as a corporate asset.

171

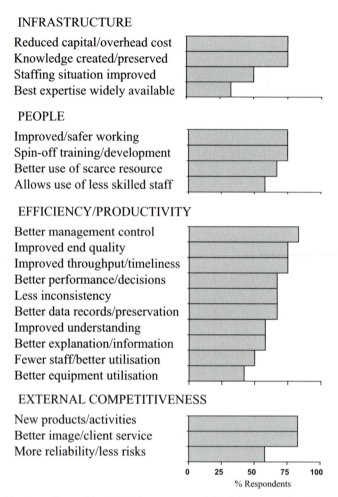

INFRASTRUCTURE
Reduced capital/overhead cost
Knowledge created/preserved
Staffing situation improved
Best expertise widely available

PEOPLE
Improved/safer working
Spin-off training/development
Better use of scarce resource
Allows use of less skilled staff

EFFICIENCY/PRODUCTIVITY
Better management control
Improved end quality
Improved throughput/timeliness
Better performance/decisions
Less inconsistency
Better data records/preservation
Improved understanding
Better explanation/information
Fewer staff/better utilisation
Better equipment utilisation

EXTERNAL COMPETITIVENESS
New products/activities
Better image/client service
More reliability/less risks

0   25   50   75   100
% Respondents

Figure 11.6 Key benefits as identified in a survey of 12 fully operational expert systems in the UK as reported by Shaw (1990)

Such is the overall picture of the benefits of expert systems in general. The question is whether or not the same applies to expert systems in the domain of product formulation. This can only be answered through a detailed examination of those systems successfully implemented where benefits have been reported (Table 11.1). Of the ten systems, three (INFORM, WOOLY and TEXPERTO) have been developed for use by customer service technicians and seven as aids for knowledgeable formulators. Benefits explicitly reported have been:

- **Knowledge protection and availability** – The existence of a coherent, durable knowledge base not affected by staff turnover. The developers of the Capsugel system have reported the benefit of being able to use knowledge from experts from many industrial companies in Europe, USA and Japan (Lai *et al.*, 1996). The developers of both the Cadila system and the Sanofi system have reported the benefit of the prompt availability of information and the rapid access to physical chemical data of both drugs and excipients reducing the time spent searching literature (Ramani *et al.*, 1992; Bateman *et al.*, 1996).

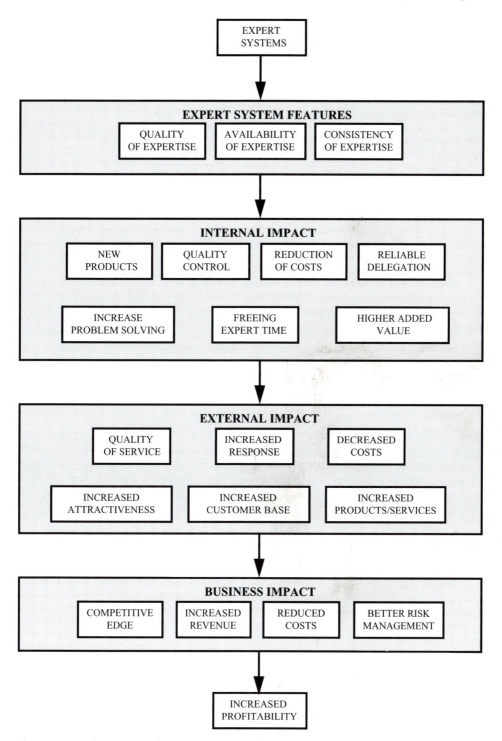

Figure 11.7   The impact of expert systems on business as reported by Thomas (1991)

Table 11.1 Product formulation expert systems used in survey to assess benefits (see Chapters 8 and 9 for details on systems)

System	Product	Organisation
INFORM	Inks	Exxon
WOOLY	Wool dyeing	Sandoz
TEXPERTO	Textile finishing	Sandoz
SOLTAN	Suncare	Boots
	Capsules	University of London/Capsugel
	Capsules	Sanofi
	Tablets	Cadila Laboratories
	Tablets	Zeneca Pharmaceuticals
	Parenterals	Zeneca Pharmaceuticals
	Tablet film coatings	Zeneca Pharmaceuticals

The instant availability of knowledge was a particular benefit noted by the developers of WOOLY and TEXPERTO since customer service technicians were then able to provide a quick response to customer queries (Frie and Walliser, 1988; Frie and Poppenwimmer, 1992).

- **Consistency** – All systems generated robust formulations with increased certainty and consistency. This was seen as a distinct benefit for systems developed in the pharmaceutical field where regulatory issues are important. It was also seen as being important in responding to customer queries (Frie and Poppenwimmer, 1992).

- **Training aid** – All systems have been used to provide training for both novice and, indeed, experienced formulators. The developers of the SOLTAN system have stated that experienced formulators use their expert systems to expose themselves to new raw material combinations with which they are not familiar. Bateman *et al.* (1996) have suggested that the documentation used in the development of the Sanofi system be adapted to train novice formulators. Frisch *et al.* (1990) have reported that INFORM has been successful as a training tool in improving effectiveness of novice formulators.

- **Speed of development** – Reduction in the duration of the formulation process has been reported by many (Wood, 1991; Frie and Poppenwimmer, 1992; Ramani *et al.*, 1992; Rowe, 1993). A rapid response to a customer query is important for customer service technicians. Wood (1991) has reported that formulators using SOLTAN can produce in 20 minutes a formulation that might otherwise have taken two days to achieve. Ramani *et al.* (1992) have reported a 35 per cent reduction in the total time needed to develop a new tablet formulation.

- **Cost savings** – Cost savings can be achieved not only by reducing the development time but also by the more effective use of materials especially if material cost and controls are included in the system. Ramani *et al.* (1992) have reported that use of their system has been a benefit in planning the purchase and stocking of excipients. The developers of SOLTAN have reported that formulations generated by their system are cost effective in terms not only of savings in raw material costs but also because fewer numbers of ingredients are used as compared to traditional formulations. Several users have also reported a decrease in the size of raw material inventories since their expert systems only use those materials specified in the database.

- **Freeing experts** – The implementation of expert systems in product formulation has inevitably allowed expert formulators to devote more time to innovation (Frisch *et al.*, 1990; Wood, 1991; Rowe, 1993). The developers of the SOLTAN system have reported that the time saved using their expert system typically releases about 30 days of formulating time per year per formulator. Of course, experienced formulators originally involved in training will also have more time to devote to innovation.

- **Improved communication** – Rowe (1993) has reported that expert systems in Zeneca Pharmaceuticals have provided a common platform from which to discuss and manage changes in working practice and to identify those critical areas requiring research and/or rationalisation. The developers of SOLTAN have reported that use of their system has made them scrutinise the way in which they formulated products highlighting shortfalls from the ideal. They also report that they have discovered previously unknown relationships between ingredients and properties in their products. The benefit of an expert system in promoting discussion has also been reported by Bateman *et al.* (1996).

Of all the systems in product formulation only one has provided costings and undertaken a cost benefit analysis. Developers of SOLTAN have estimated the overall cost of their system to be £10 400 for hardware and software, £6000 for consultancy and £9000 for expert's time making a total of £25 400. Annual cost savings in the region of £200 000 have been reported delivering a payback of approximately three months.

It is interesting to note that where expert systems have been implemented in product formulation early scepticism among potential users has generally changed to a mood of enthusiastic participation. It is unlikely that expert systems will ever replace expert formulators but as a decision support tool they are invaluable, delivering many benefits both measurable and intangible.

11.3   Neural Networks/Genetic Algorithms

Just as expert systems allow companies to capitalise and control the use and reuse of knowledge and expertise, neural networks and genetic algorithms allow companies to capitalise and control the use and reuse of data, often a hard earned and under valued asset.

Turban (1995) has listed the benefits of the technology to include:

- Pattern recognition especially in situations where rules are unknown.
- Generalisation in that neural networks can be used to analyse noisy and incomplete data.
- Fault tolerance in that damage to a few neurons or links within the network does not bring it to a halt.
- Adaptability and flexibility in that as a database expands the network can be easily retrained.
- Rapid response in that neural networks, once trained, are very fast.

In an overview of neural computing (DTI, 1993) it was claimed that the introduction of neural computing can yield benefits in a number of areas:

- improved accuracy and system performance;
- ability to automate previously manual processes;
- reduced development times;

although no data were given to support these claims.

Recently an extensive survey of the use of neural computing applications in UK companies covering all business sectors has been reported (Rees, 1996). Fifty-one potential users (i.e. organisations considering the implementation of one or more neural computing systems in the following two years) and 75 current users of the technology were asked to rate the benefits they either hoped to realise or had achieved according to a scale from 1 to 5 with 1 being no benefit and 5 being a major benefit. The results are shown in Figure 11.8. It can be seen that the current users obtained a wide range of benefits from their applications with the major ones being improved quality, improved response times and increased quality. The benefits are very similar to those for expert systems (Figures 11.3 and 11.6), which is not surprising given the close relationship between data and knowledge (Figure 2.3).

In general the potential users had slightly higher expectations than those realised by the users but the two sets of ratings are very close, suggesting that the potential users do have realistic expectations of the perceived benefits. It is interesting to note that when the current users were asked how satisfied they were with their neural computing systems, 84 per cent replied that they were either satisfied or very satisfied with their applications. Only 3 per cent were dissatisfied although 13 per cent did not express an opinion (Figure 11.9).

An analysis of the benefits seen on using neural networks and genetic algorithms for modelling and optimising formulations for the applications discussed in Chapter 10 reveals the following:

- Effective use of incomplete data sets.
- Rapid analysis of data.
- Relatively easy to retrain network to accommodate more data.
- Effective explanation of the total design space irrespective of the complexity of interaction between the ingredients of the formulation.
- Ability to accommodate constraints and preferences allowing a number of optimised formulations to be developed.
- Reduction in experimentation.

VerDuin (1995) in his book *Better Products Faster* has extrapolated these benefits in a business context to include:

- Enhancement of product quality and performance at lower cost.
- Shorter time to market.
- Development of new products and processes.
- Improved responses to customer demands.
- Improved processing efficiency.
- Improved confidence.
- Increased competitive edge.

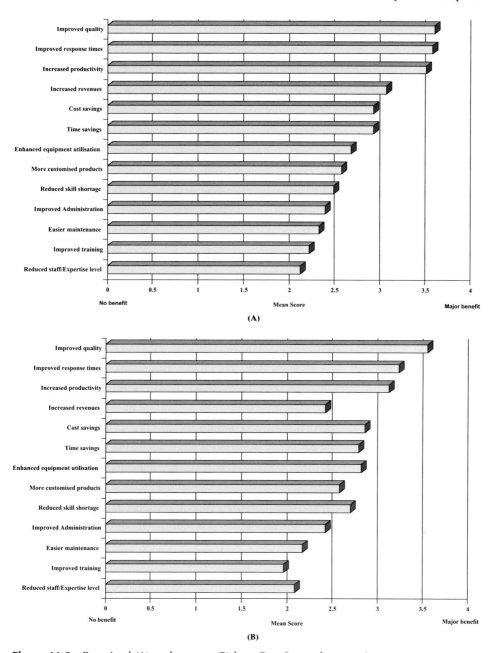

Figure 11.8 Perceived (A) and proven (B) benefits of neural computing systems as identified in a survey of potential and current users in the UK as reported by Rees (1996)

In a detailed analysis of two applications implemented with CAD/Chem from AI Ware Inc., ignoring savings in facilities costs and benefits from faster time to market, VerDuin (1995) has estimated a payback of between three and eight months. It would appear that many companies are now using this software for modelling and optimising formulations (Table 10.1) but only a few appear willing to reveal their experiences.

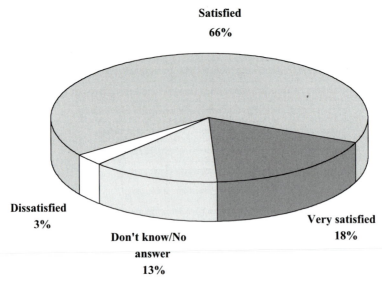

Satisfied
66%

Dissatisfied
3%

Don't know/No
answer
13%

Very satisfied
18%

Figure 11.9 User satisfaction with neural computing applications in the UK as reported by Rees (1996)

11.4 Conclusion

As can be seen, there are measurable benefits in implementing both expert systems and neural networks/genetic algorithms although intangible benefits abound. The question is how can senior management decide whether or not their business would benefit from implementation. Generalisation is difficult, but Thomas (1991) has suggested that the key factor for expert system implementation is the existence of costly expertise bottlenecks i.e. recurrent business problems where solution relies on the application of scarce expertise. He has suggested that such a bottleneck would have to cost the company at least £50 000 pa before it is worth considering implementation. This was a generalisation for all expert systems. Experience in the product formulation domain would suggest that this figure could be reduced by as much as half to £25 000 pa. Applying the same argument to neural networks where the cost of development and implementation is minimal (only training is required to use the software) even this figure could be very much reduced, possibly by as much as a factor of five. In these cases payback will be within a year of implementation.

Intelligent software should now be viewed as an important weapon in the armoury of senior management. The technology is now mature and has proved its ability to generate real business benefit. Expert systems and neural networks/genetic algorithms should be considered routinely as one of the methods available in increasing competitive edge.

References

BATEMAN, S.D., VERLIN, J., RUSSO, M., GUILLOT, M. and LAUGHLIN, S.M., 1996, The development and validation of a capsule formulation knowledge-based system, *Pharm. Technol.*, **20** (3) 174–184.

Dewar, J., 1989, Expert system trends revealed, *Systems International*, **17** (7), 12–14.

DTI, 1993, *Best Practice Guidelines for Developing Neural Computing Applications – An Overview*, London: DTI.

Frie, G. and Poppenwimmer, K., 1992, TEXPERTO – ein expertensystem fur die ausrustung, *Textilveredlung*, **27**, 276–279.

Frie, G. and Walliser, R., 1988, WOOLY – ein expertensystem fur den wollfarber, *Textilveredlung*, **23**, 203–205.

Frisch, P.D., Lalka, G.J. and Orrick, J.F., 1990, INFORM – a generalised ink formulation assistant, *American Ink Maker*, **68** (10), 56–68.

Lai, S., Podczeck, F., Newton, J.M. and Daumesnil, R., 1996, An expert system to aid the development of capsule formulations, *Pharm. Tech. Eur.*, **8** (9), 60–68.

Ramani, K.V., Patel, M.R. and Patel, S.K., 1992, An expert system for drug preformulation in a pharmaceutical company, *Interfaces*, **22** (2), 101–108.

Rees, C., 1996, *Neural Computing – Learning Solutions, User survey*, London: DTI.

Rowe, R.C., 1993, An expert system for the formulation of pharmaceutical tablets, *Manufacturing Intelligence*, **14**, 13–15.

Shaw, R., 1990, *Expert System Opportunities, Guidelines for the Introduction of Expert Systems Technology*, London: HMSO.

Thomas, M., 1991, How should senior managers react to expert systems, *Manufacturing Intelligence*, **7**, 6–8.

Tinsley, H., 1992, Expert systems in manufacturing, an overview, *Manufacturing Intelligence*, **9**, 7–9.

Turban, E., 1995, *Decision Support Systems and Expert Systems*, Englewood Cliffs, NJ: Prentice-Hall.

VerDuin, W.H., 1995, *Better Products Faster*, New York: Irwin.

Wood, M., 1991, Expert systems save formulation time, *Lab-Equipment Digest*, December, 17–19.

12

Issues and Limitations of Intelligent Software

12.1 Introduction

The potential of intelligent software such as expert systems and neural networks/ genetic algorithms to solve all business problems should not be overstated. These are a cost effective way of solving certain classes of problems but there are several issues and limitations that have slowed down their acceptance. Some of these have been highlighted in the Systems International/es (Connect) survey of expert systems applications (Dewar, 1989). The key factors which prevented implementation (Figure 12.1) tended to be those that indicated that the budget holder was not prepared to commit resources, mainly because management could not be convinced of the benefits. The least important factors were those related to the personnel (i.e. the user or expert) resources. A shortage of knowledge engineers was cited as a constraint in the early stages of development but less so at later stages. Maintenance was identified as an issue in another section of the survey (Dewar, 1989). In another survey, this time involving small/medium companies in the manufacturing and process industries in the UK, the main concern about implementing an expert system was the cost of its development and subsequent maintenance (Tinsley, 1992).

Similar issues, this time in applications of neural networks, have also been identified in a recent survey of 75 users, with 93 applications, in a wide range of industrial sectors in the UK (Rees, 1996). Respondents were asked to identify areas where they had experienced problems from a list of potential problem areas. Their replies (Figure 12.2) showed the general level of problems identified to be relatively low; 39 per cent of applications had experienced problems as a result of lack of data with other major problem areas being related to software and lack of development skills. A total of 22 per cent experienced problems with methodology but only 12 per cent identified lack of support from management as a problem. The latter figure is comparable with that experienced for expert systems (Figure 12.1).

All of these and other issues are discussed in this chapter under the broad headings of Technical issues and Organisational issues.

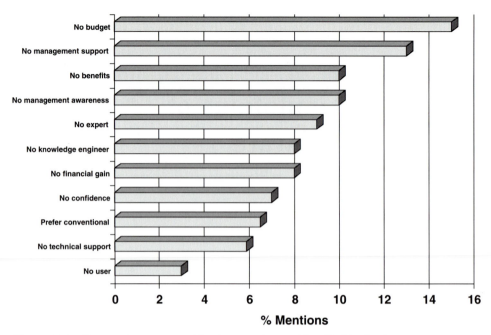

Figure 12.1 Factors that prevented implementation as identified in the Systems International/es (Connect) survey of expert systems applications as reported by Dewar (1989)

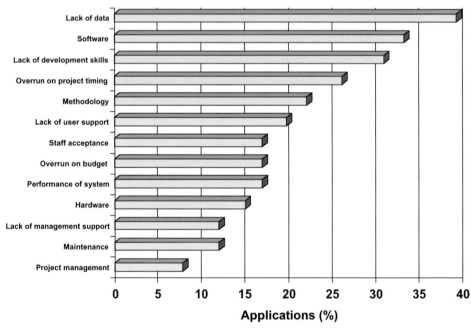

Figure 12.2 Problem areas identified by users of neural networks as reported by Rees (1996)

12.2 Technical Issues

Included under this heading are the identification of potential applications, choice of software, verification and validation, and maintenance and refinement of the applications.

12.2.1 *Application Identification*

Without the potential to deliver real business benefit, management cannot be expected to support or resource projects and hence the identification of the right application is an essential prerequisite in the implementation of intelligent software. The question to be asked is not where intelligent software can be used in the business but where the business could use intelligent software. The fact that other methods are not appropriate for the application does not mean that intelligent software is necessary to solve the problem. Expert systems and neural networks/genetic algorithms each require a number of technical features that are not normally a feature of conventional computing. If the candidate application does not possess these features then intelligent software may not be the appropriate solution.

Features which indicate applications where expert systems may provide an advantage (Shaw, 1990; Turban, 1995) are:

- The application should be primarily symbolic in structure.
- The application should be rule-based and heuristics should be available for solution.
- The application should have a reasonable degree of complexity which is neither too easy nor too difficult.
- The application should be of a manageable size. If too large it should be able to be easily subdivided into manageable modules.
- At least one expert who is both co-operative and articulate should be available.
- The application should involve the analysis of a range of options and non-optimal results can be tolerated.
- Rapid repeated decision making of a trivial nature is required.

Features which indicate applications where neural networks/genetic algorithms may provide an advantage are:

- The application should be primarily numeric in structure.
- Large quantities of data should be available.
- The application should deal with poor quality or incomplete data not amenable to statistical analysis.
- The application should be multi-dimensional where it is difficult to specify a model for mathematical simulation.
- It should be difficult to specify rules.
- The application needs to be adaptive when new data become available.

It should be noted that if there are doubts about the availability of data the application should not proceed since lack of suitable data is one of the main causes for failure in neural network projects (Rees, 1996).

For both cases the application should always:

- be of practical importance;
- meet a real business need;
- be part of an essential activity;
- occur in a stable environment.

Experience in the domain of product formulation would suggest that these features are very good pointers to a successful implementation and should be adopted as a screening process for assessing the technical feasibility of an application.

Since a first time intelligent software project is likely to be high profile and failure will be very visible, a poor choice of application can have disastrous consequences not least in the outright rejection of the technology. Attempting to develop an application that will do everything in the first instance can be just as bad. It is better either to limit the scope of the application at the outset, or subdivide the application domain into smaller manageable modules and then develop each module in turn. Both these approaches have proved successful in developing expert systems for formulating aluminium alloys where the initial scope was limited in size (Rychener *et al.*, 1985) and pharmaceuticals where the domain was divided into different formulation types (Stricker *et al.*, 1994). Experience has shown that generally the quality of the performance of the divided system is more important than the scope of the application. This does not mean that toy (trivial) applications should be developed since these will rapidly lose credibility and support from both experts and management.

There are no hard and fast rules as to what makes a good application but it can be guaranteed that, if everything falls into place, any early scepticism among experts and management will rapidly change to enthusiastic participation.

12.2.2 *Software Selection*

Software selection is complex, not least because of the large number of software packages on the market. There are many generic issues involved in the selection of suitable software:

- Applicability – suitability of tool to the domain.
- Flexibility – ability to adapt to different domains.
- Extendibility – ability to be extended by the addition of new components e.g. user interface.
- Portability – ability to be transferred to different hardware.
- Interconnectivity – ability to be integrated with other software packages e.g. databases.
- Efficiency – ability to provide good performance.
- Operability – ease of use.
- Security – ability to be protected against unauthorised access.
- Reliability – ability to perform according to specification.
- Maintainability – ability to be easily maintained.

- Size – reference to size of knowledge base or amount of data to be processed.
- Richness – reference to varieties of knowledge representation techniques, reasoning methods, etc. for expert systems; reference to library of network architectures and training algorithms for neural networks.
- Cost – including licences, updates, support, training and other indirect costs.
- Reputation – known reputation of vendor, consultancy, etc.

In-depth evaluations of software packages often appear in computer magazines but these are often subjective and the capabilities of the packages change regularly due to the release of new versions.

In the case of expert systems there are a plethora of software ranging from conventional languages through to special purpose languages, environments and shells/tools (Chapter 2). It is interesting to look at the distribution of the types of software used to develop expert systems. The results of three surveys are given in Figure 12.3. The first survey (Figure 12.3A) is one carried out in 1988 and reported by Edwards (1991). It shows the distribution of software for 405 expert systems which had been reported as reaching at least field trial stage by the end of 1988. The second (Figure 12.3B) is based on 12 successfully implemented industrial expert systems reported by the Department of Trade and Industry (DTI) in 1990 (Shaw, 1990). The third (Figure 12.3C) has been collated by the authors for the specific domain of product formulation. It is based on 27 expert systems, data being extracted from the literature and personal knowledge. It can be seen that, in all three surveys, the majority of expert systems have been developed using shells or domain specific tools with only a quarter to a third being developed using languages. The large percentage of shells/tools used for product formulation is due to the inclusion of the domain specific tool PFES (Chapter 3) which is now being used extensively in the development of expert systems in this domain.

Because of the task structure in formulation expert systems (Bold, 1989) a certain functionality of the software is desirable. As part of the Alvey Project to investigate knowledge-based systems for product formulation, the team identified a number of requirements that need to be supported (Alvey, 1987):

- Specification of the formulation problem. This may need to be modified during the course of the formulation process.
- Formulation from first principles.
- Modification of the formulation. The system should assist the formulator to modify a partial or complete formulation to meet some aspect of the problem specification.
- Searching/retrieval for similar past formulations. This is especially helpful if there are historical formulations held in an existing computer system.
- Selection of topic to address. The system should assist the formulator to decide which aspect of the formulation problem to work on. This requires an analysis and comparison of the current state of the proposed formulation with the specification.
- Support for the explanation of different formulation routes and allowing the formulator to change the course of the process.
- Prediction of test results.
- Assessing the requirements for testing.

A

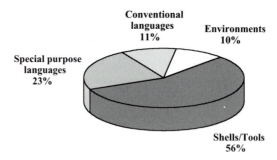

B

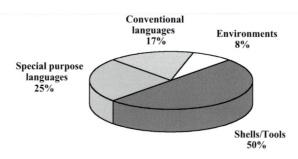

C

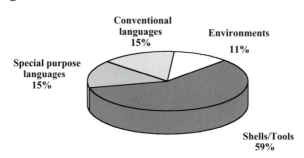

Figure 12.3 Distribution of development tools used for expert systems: A, data from 1988 for 405 systems (Edwards, 1991); B, data from 1990 for 12 systems (Shaw, 1990); C, data from 27 product formulatuon expert systems (Rowe and Roberts, unpublished data)

- Acceptance of test results.
- Support for the evolution of knowledge. The system should assist the formulator to update the knowledge base.
- Flexibility of control. The formulator can either maintain complete control or relinquish it to a chosen degree.
- Interconnectivity to external databases and mathematical models and simulations.
- Explanation of decisions and the factors the system took into account in arriving at the recommendation.

- Revision support. The system should allow the formulator to revise decisions.

- Monitoring facilities. The system should keep the formulator informed of progress on the formulation process.

- Suspension facilities. The system should allow the formulator to save the state of progress (e.g. while awaiting test results) and, on resumption, replay the actions taken so far.

Ideally all these requirements should be accommodated by the software chosen for any problem in the domain of product formulation. However, it may well be that certain requirements do not need to be addressed for specific problems e.g. in developing a system for an initial formulation without any need for reformulation, the software would not be required to support any facilities for assessing the requirement for testing or the acceptance of test results. The only software with the majority of these facilities inbuilt is the domain specific tool PFES (Chapter 3).

For applications involving the use of neural networks/genetic algorithms, the selection of software is not quite as difficult as it is for expert systems. Here the primary question is one of whether or not to use an entry level package or a project development package. The former provides facilities for experimenting with and gaining an understanding of the basic concepts; generally they are inexpensive, support only multilayer perceptron (MLP) architecture and are simple to use. The latter provide more advanced features and are designed for the development and delivery of complete neural computing applications; generally they are more expensive and tend to support a variety of network architectures and training algorithms. They also allow editing, pre- and post-processing of data and in some cases generate implementation code. In many areas entry level packages can compete favourably with software costing much more. In addition some entry level packages can be easily upgraded to more advanced versions providing a secondary path from entry level to advanced functionality.

An analysis of the applications in Chapter 10 shows that all could be modelled using the multilayer perceptron, many with only one hidden layer. The majority were developed using either a project development package or the domain specific tool CAD/Chem (Chapter 6).

General experience with the two domain specific tools – PFES for expert systems and CAD/Chem for neural networks/genetic algorithms – would suggest that their use results in the rapid development of useful, cost effective applications. Because their functionality has been specifically designed to suit the domain of product formulation they tend to be more acceptable to formulators and management. There is more enthusiastic participation of formulators, with the result that applications developed with these tools are used and do not get terminated.

12.2.3 *Verification and Validation*

Whether or not any application developed using intelligent software is ultimately used in an organisation depends on establishing and maintaining the confidence of the users in its performance. For an expert system the users must be convinced that it produces results of the same quality/reliability as those produced by the domain expert while for neural networks/genetic algorithms the users must be convinced

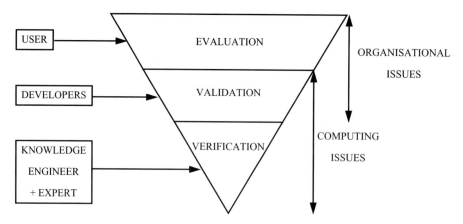

Figure 12.4 Relationships between evaluation, validation and verification and the issues involved

that the model correctly predicts the output for both known and unknown inputs covering the complete design space.

Since in developing applications using intelligent software it is the human cognitive activities that are being modelled, the evaluation of the performance of the system must include concepts beyond the purely mechanical replication of certain requirements. In this respect evaluation is the highest level concept and the broadest dealing with the contributions of the application towards the success of the organisation. Evaluation includes validation which deals with the performance of the system (i.e. substantiating whether or not the system has attained an adequate level of performance with an acceptable level of accuracy and reliability), and verification which deals with the construction of the system (i.e. substantiating whether or not the system correctly implements its specification). In other words verification confirms that the system has been constructed correctly while validation confirms that the correct system has been constructed. Although complimentary these concepts are different. There are many examples of applications which have been developed as per specification but did not function in practice because certain elements were absent and hence failed in validation. Similarly some applications may be valid but unable to be used by the organisation because of circumstances not directly related to it (e.g. the unexpected retirement of the product champion). These concepts of evaluation, validation and verification can be viewed as shown schematically in Figure 12.4.

Verification and validation achieve their objectives using a combination of three types of analysis:

- Static analysis or the manual or automatic examination of the information contained in the system which does not involve execution of the application.
- Dynamic analysis or the evaluation of the functionality of the system which does involve execution of the application.
- Formal analysis which is the evaluation of the symbolic execution of the system using mathematical techniques.

Verification applies to all components of the developed system and is best carried out by the knowledge engineer and expert. For instance, in the application of the knowledge the developers would use static testing to check the consistency, corrections and completeness of the knowledge therein as well as checking for redundant, conflicting and circular rules. For verifying the inference engine and reasoning process the developers would use dynamic testing to see if the system produced correct answers.

In validation dynamic analysis is used to compare the performance of the system using test cases for expert systems and test data for neural networks. These can be chosen at random or by various experts (often called black box testing) or by using representative examples (often called white box testing). The performance can be judged either qualitatively using subjective measures or quantitatively using statistical measures. The latter is always used for neural networks while the former is often used for expert systems. Common approaches to qualitative validation are:

- Face validation where an appraisal is carried out by the developers and potential users to assess the credibility of the result.
- Predictive validation where historic test cases are used and the results are compared.
- Turing testing where a blind comparison is made between the results from the expert system and the results from a human expert on the same set of test cases.
- Field testing where the expert system is placed in its operational environment and the user performs live testing.

Currently the verification and validation of expert systems is informal, subjective, time-consuming, tedious, and arbitrary (Smith and Kandel, 1993). A major issue is the lack of resources with validation being allocated significantly less of the total budget than planned. In addition validation efforts are often driven by the production life cycle and further developments and enhancements are perceived as being more important (Medsker and Liebowitz, 1994). For a comprehensive treatise on verification and validation of rule-based expert systems the reader is referred to Smith and Kandel (1993).

In the domain of product formulation only one group, Bateman *et al.* (1996), has specifically reported a verification and validation protocol. Although the authors used 40 test cases to validate their system for capsule formulation, no performance criteria were given. Judging the quality of formulations and measuring real differences is a specific issue in this domain. There is an opinion that the provision of a reasonable initial formulation which could be further refined, if required, is the best that can be achieved but many would argue against this approach.

Verification and validation of applications developed using intelligent software remains a contentious issue. There is undoubtedly a need for more standards and methodologies and it is essential that more resources are allocated to this area. If at all possible it is best to verify and validate small parts of the system as they are being implemented since this will dramatically reduce the complexity of the validation of the final system.

12.2.4 *Maintenance and Refinement*

The need for maintenance and refinement is motivated by the critically important reason to ensure a long operational life for the application as this will improve the chances of the system returning the benefits as listed in Chapter 11. Applications often fail, due to the emergence of errors that have not been identified elsewhere, to changes in the environment or to the introduction of new user requirements. The goals of maintenance and refinement are thus:

- correcting errors and bugs;
- updating the system in order to meet changes in hardware and software;
- progressively updating the system as a result of evolving needs and knowledge drift.

Maintenance can absorb a large proportion of the life time cost of an operational system; estimates are usually over 50 per cent and can run as high as 80 per cent (Edwards, 1991).

Correcting errors in the rule-base of an expert system triggered when test cases are wrongly solved during validation is known as knowledge refinement. Traditionally this has been identified as a subset of knowledge acquisition but recently it has been argued that it should be thought of as complimenting verification and validation (Craw, 1996). A refinement tool which is currently being developed to automate this process is KRUST (Knowledge Refinement Using Semantic Trees). The operation of KRUST may be broken down into three tasks:

- Blame allocation which determines which rule or parts of rules might be responsible for the error.
- Refinement generation which suggests modifications that may correct the error.
- Refinement selections which select the best of the possible refinements according to some criteria.

KRUST is supplied with a set of training examples. Figure 12.5 shows KRUST using one training example at a time to generate refinements while the remaining examples are used to filter these refinements (Craw and Sleeman, 1995).

KRUST has recently been applied to refining an expert system for formulating tablets using PFES (Chapter 3) and found to be successful in identifying and refining faults for incorrect filler, incorrect quantity of binder and multiple faults in specification (Boswell *et al.*, 1996, 1997).

Compensation for knowledge drift over time is an important goal for maintenance of expert systems. Very few fields involving experts remain static and hence knowledge bases and inference mechanisms will need to be continually under review to ensure that the application does not become outmoded. Both Rowe (1993) and Lai *et al.* (1996) have reported their experiences of this problem for expert systems for formulating tablets and capsules respectively.

Rowe (1993) used consultancy support to upgrade the Zeneca system after identifying with management and experts the new philosophy to be adopted for the upgrade. Lai *et al.* (1996) reported a process whereby feedback reports from users were analysed by the developers of the system and possible changes to the knowledge base implemented. They also reported a semi-automatic process by which the system monitors user habits and collects data about the use of excipients. The data are then statistically evaluated and any changes authorised by the developers. Annual meetings are used to discuss refinements and enhancements.

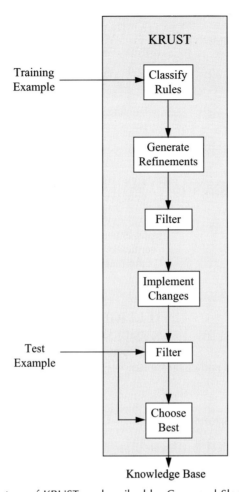

Figure 12.5 The structure of KRUST as described by Craw and Sleeman (1995)

It is important to define a strategy for maintenance and refinement since it is inevitable that they will need to be done. Maintenance and refinement are never complete; they continue as long as the application is being used. For a comprehensive treatise on the theory, techniques and tools for maintaining knowledge-based systems the reader is referred to Cohen and Bench-Capon (1993).

12.3 Organisational Issues

Although developing applications based on intelligent software may involve sizeable initial and ongoing costs, many organisations take unnecessary risks and fail to produce a usable system. Generally this is not primarily due to technical issues not being adhered to but is due to organisational difficulties not being foreseen. Some of these, for example, lack of management support, problems with budget, and staff acceptance have already been highlighted as issues in Figures 12.1 and 12.2. These and others are addressed under the headings of staff roles and responsibilities, development strategy, financial considerations, security and project planning/ management.

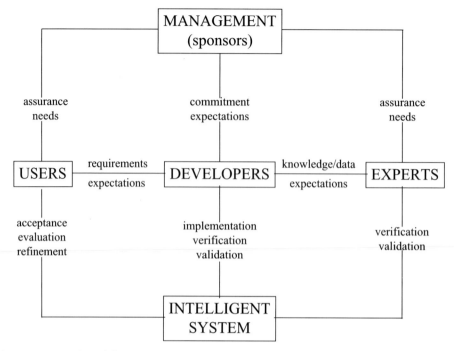

Figure 12.6 Roles of the participants in the development of intelligent systems and their interactions

12.3.1 *Roles and Responsibilities*

When initiating a project to develop an application using intelligent software, everybody in the organisation needs to understand what the project is, its aims, how it is going to be undertaken and the roles and responsibilities of the participants. This means that management has a pivotal role in the project:

- to determine whether or not there exist problems with the business to which intelligent software offers the best solution;
- to direct and resource an initiative;
- to insist that a business focus is maintained;
- to insist that the project is cost effective.

Managers do not need to have an in-depth knowledge of the technology but their role should be one of devil's advocate. Management should be convinced that:

- the project is business driven rather than technology driven;
- the technology chosen is the best and most cost-effective for the project;
- software compatibility is maintained.

Hence the management role is crucial to the success of the project. Indeed, it is now known from studies that organisations which are successful in developing intelligent systems are those whose management plays an active role in steering and backing their initiatives. Essentially management sets the framework within which the developers work. Management sponsors of the project initiate work based on the perceived needs of the users and experts (Figure 12.6). Its commitment is essential but it needs to have assurances that the application under development is indeed required.

The developers liaise with the users and experts to ascertain the requirements of the application to acquire the knowledge and or/data. They also manage the expectations of the other participants. Verification and validation of the developed system is made both by the developers and experts.

The experts, being the sources of the knowledge/data must be prepared to co-operate with the developers. In addition, they must be committed to the success of the project and be able to work closely with the developer to create, verify and validate the final system.

The users must be involved at the outset, not only in setting the requirements but also in defining goals. They are also involved in the later stages of development evaluating the developed system and suggesting improvements.

It is important at the outset to identify the participants filling each of the roles. Indeed more than one role could be filled by a single person. However, in some cases, several people could be involved in the same role e.g. multiple experts for knowledge acquisition. Each project will be different and there are no hard and fast rules regarding the composition of the project team. Many systems have been successfully produced by two person teams centred around the roles of knowledge engineer and user/expert.

An issue that must be sensitively managed at the outset is that of the role of the expert and users after implementation of the intelligent systems. Although in all the surveys (Figures 11.3 and 11.8) reduced staffing has generally been seen as the least important benefit of implementation, it can still be an issue with some individuals. It is inevitable that there will be a change in the job content of both the expert and the users, which may or may not result in increased opportunities for promotion and development. If it is seen by individuals that implementation of a system will, in any way, adversely affect status or career pathways, the result will be lack of co-operation not only at the development stage but also after implementation. In these situations it is essential that management motivates and encourages the participants involved.

12.3.2 *Development Strategy*

To derive maximum business benefit from intelligent systems an organisation must be confident that it is developing them in the most effective way with the right infrastructure and resources. There are three principle strategies that can be applied:

- In-house or 'do it yourself' – this course of action is attractive for those organisations that already possess the skills and resources necessary. It is specifically attractive to those companies that want to develop applications containing significant levels of proprietary or sensitive knowledge/data. It is not an attractive option for small companies wanting to develop a small number of applications as the ongoing costs of maintaining a central resource can be prohibitive.

- Consultancy – this is an attractive option for those organisations that do not have, or cannot afford, the necessary expertise in-house but want to have control over the development of their applications.

- Joint venture with either a software vendor or an academic institution. This course of action is ideal for those organisations that cannot afford the necessary expertise but want to test the feasibility of certain options.

All of these strategies have been applied in the development of successful applications in the domain of product formulation (Chapters 8, 9 and 10). It is difficult to define hard and fast rules as to which strategy is the best. Each application must be considered on merit and management needs to ensure that the investment is justified in light of the perceived benefits. The strategy chosen will certainly have an impact on budgets.

12.3.3 *Financial Considerations*

Committing the right level of resource is essential if an intelligent system is to be successful. Implementation costs can be divided into two distinct groups: direct costs which involve the costs of labour and equipment (software, hardware, etc.); and indirect costs which include the cost of training and maintenance. The latter are often difficult to predict at the outset of the project and are often ignored. However, as pointed out by Edwards (1991) maintenance can absorb a large proportion of the lifetime cost of an operational expert system.

Direct costs will be dependent on the size of the application developed and hence are difficult to generalise. For costings on specific expert systems successfully implemented in the UK the reader is referred to the 12 case studies reported by the Department of Trade and Industry (Shaw, 1990).

Unfortunately there are very few costings for applications in the domain of product formulation. To the author's knowledge data are available on only one – an expert system developed by personnel from the Boots Company Ltd UK and Logica UK Ltd for the formulation of suncare products. In this case the direct costs were (Wood, 1991):

Equipment costs (hardware and software)	£10 400
Consultancy	£6 000
Formulators	£9 000
Total	£25 400

It is interesting to note that consultancy costs were approximately £300 per man day and labour costs for formulators approximately £150 per man day.

With neural network applications, in addition to the direct costs of labour and equipment, there will be specific costs associated with the data generation/collection especially if it is to be collected from plant machinery or requires reformatting from another computerised system. In addition, data collection systems can take a considerable time to perfect. Two areas in neural computing projects carry extra risks:

- There are often cost or time resources associated with data generation/collection.
- There are often performance shortfalls because of the difficulty in estimating performance at the outset.

Both can lead to increased development times and hence cost.

In order to minimise cost and risk, Thomas (1991) has suggested that any investment be managed by:

- Use of 'off the shelf' rather than bespoke software since this is likely to involve lower direct costs, have lower risk of failure and hence be more cost effective.
- Undertake phased rather than large implementation since this reduces risks and allows benefits to flow earlier.
- Build utility rather than luxury systems since these will be less expensive and handling the core of a problem usually maximises the return on investment.

Although these suggestions were aimed at potential developers of expert systems in a time of recession, they are generally applicable to the development of any intelligent software.

12.3.4 *Security*

One of the most overlooked issues in intelligent software is security. The knowledge in an expert system or data in a neural network model may well be valuable to competitors and must be kept secure. This is best done by password protection operated at several levels:

Low: run the application by the user.

Medium: browse the knowledge base (specific to expert systems).

High: allow editing, maintenance and refinement.

Embodied knowledge and data can also be protected using encryption of the application files. Appropriate back-up copies of the application should exist and be properly stored. Knowledge and data are both hard earned assets and, although often undervalued, must be kept secure.

12.3.5 *Project Planning/Management*

There are several critical success factors for a successful application of intelligent software:

- There is a real business need with quantifiable benefits.
- The application is suitable.
- The correct technology is chosen.
- The project team is strong and committed.
- A prototype showing real functionality can be built rapidly.

Most of these factors could be applied to any project. In other words, intelligent software projects are not very different from any other project and can be planned and managed using common practices. There are many methodologies in the literature (e.g. Edwards, 1991; Guida and Tasso, 1994) with guidelines issued by the DTI for both expert systems and neural networks (Shaw, 1990; DTI, 1994). All follow a similar life cycle:

- Project proposal/definition – in this phase it is necessary to identify the business need, develop a vision and conduct a feasibility study thus producing a business case that will support the investment in developing the application.

- Design and development – in this phase an iterative approach is used to build the application. Probably the most well established approach is that of rapid prototyping. This allows design decisions to be resolved through experimentation and provides a number of other benefits: experiments can be easily performed on a subsystem of the design; different hardware and software can be easily tested; and the process provides early feedback to the project team allowing reflection and review if performance is not what was intended.

- Testing and evaluation – this phase is very important in convincing the users of the quality and reliability of the application. It also allows decisions to be made regarding plans for implementation within the business e.g. the training needs of the users, type and amount of documentation required, and maintenance issues.

- Implementation – the most important objective of this phase is to ensure acceptance and use by potential users and to review the benefits against the original project objectives.

Unfortunately very little data exist either on the proportion or duration of each phase, since in many projects involving intelligent software the phases are often indistinct and overlapping. Typical values for the proportion of each phase in expert system projects (Shaw, 1990) are project definition, 10 per cent; design and prototyping, 60 per cent; and testing and evaluation, 30 per cent. In an analysis of 12 fully operational expert systems in manufacturing, engineering, medical and finance, Shaw (1990) found the duration range of project phases was:

- Feasibility – 1–12 months
- Prototyping – 1–3 months
- System design – 3–8 months
- Testing – 1–3 months
- Implementation – 3–12 months

It is interesting to note that Shaw (1990) found little use of formal design methods in these case studies. Only a few had used project planning/management systems and several confessed to serious underestimation of the various project phases. In a larger survey of expert system applications involving nearly 450 responses from a wide variety of organisations from all sectors of business in the UK it was found that barely 20 per cent of respondents had used any project planning/management systems (Dewar, 1989).

No comparable data exist for neural networks. However in a recent survey of 93 applications, from 75 current users of the technology, from a wide range of businesses in the UK, Rees (1996) found that in 57 per cent of the applications development time was less than 12 months (Figure 12.7). This shortened development time compared to that for expert systems is only to be expected because of the known problems and issues around knowledge acquisition. No details were given regarding the use of project planning/management systems.

It is essential that, in order to derive maximum benefit from the technology, all projects must be properly planned and managed. For a comprehensive treatise on

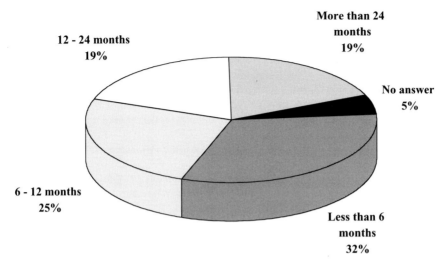

Figure 12.7 Length of development time of neural network applications as reported by Rees (1996)

the design and development of expert systems using a process model that clearly distinguishes between the primary, supporting and management processes the reader is referred to Guida and Tasso (1994). Two very useful texts are the guidelines issued by the DTI for both expert systems (Shaw, 1990) and neural networks (DTI, 1994).

12.4 Conclusion

Although there are many issues and constraints surrounding the development of applications using intelligent software, the majority can be minimised by good management. An awareness of the issues at an early stage of development of the application is essential if the project is to be successfully completed. Good preparation includes the formation of a well motivated team under the direction of a supportive and committed management and the judicious selection of a suitable application area and development tool.

References

ALVEY PROJECT REPORT, 1987, IKBS/052, *Product Formulation Expert System*, Vol. 5, Recommended Applications Methodology, London: DTI.

BATEMAN, S.D., VERLIN, J., RUSSO, M., GUILLOT, M. and LAUGHLIN, S.M., 1996, The development and validation of a capsule formulation knowledge-based system, *Pharm. Technol.*, **20** (3), 174–184.

BOLD, K., 1989, Expertensysteme unterstutzen bei der Produktformulierung, *Chem. Ztg.*, **113**, 343–346.

BOSWELL, R., CRAW, S. and ROWE, R.C., 1996, Refinement of a product formulation expert system, *Proc. ECAI–96 Workshop on Validation, Verification and Refinement of KBS*, pp. 74–79.

BOSWELL, R., CRAW, S. and ROWE, R.C., 1997, Knowledge refinement for a design system, *Proc. European Knowledge Acquisition Workshop EKAW-97*.

COHEN, F. and BENCH-CAPON, T., 1993, *Maintenance of Knowledge-Based Systems – Theory, Techniques and Tools*, London: Academic Press.

CRAW, S., 1996, Refinement complements verification and validation, *Int. J. Human-Computer Studies*, **44**, 245–256.

CRAW, S. and SLEEMAN, D., 1995, Refinement in response to validation, *Expert Systems with Applications*, **8** (3), 343–349.

DEWAR, J., 1989, Expert system trends revealed, *Systems International*, **17** (7), 12–14.

DTI (1994), *Best Practice Guidelines for Developing Neural Computing Applications*, London: DTI.

EDWARDS, J.S., 1991, *Building Knowledge-Based Systems: Towards a Methodology*, London: Pitman Publishing.

GUIDA, G. and TASSO, C., 1994, *Design and Development of Knowledge-Based Systems from Life Cycle to Methodology*, Chichester: John Wiley and Sons.

LAI, S., PODCZECK, F., NEWTON, J.M. and DAUMESNIL, R., 1996, An expert system to aid the development of capsule formulations, *Pharm. Tech. Eur.*, **8** (9), 60–68.

MEDSKER, L. and LIEBOWITZ, J., 1994, *Design and Development of Expert Systems and Neural Networks*, New York: Macmillan.

REES, C., 1996, *Neural Computing – Learning Solutions, User Survey*, London: DTI.

ROWE, R.C., 1993, An expert system for the formulation of pharmaceutical tablets, *Manufacturing Intelligence*, **14**, 13–15.

RYCHENER, M.D., FARINACCI, M.L., HULTHAGE, I. and FOX, M.S., 1985, Integration of multiple knowledge sources in ALADIN, an alloy design system, *IEEE J. Engng.*, 878–882.

SHAW, R., 1990, *Expert System Opportunities – Case Studies*, London: HMSO.

SMITH, S. and KANDEL, A., 1993, *Verification and Validation of Rule-Based Expert Systems*, Boca Raton, FL: CRC Press.

STRICKER, H., FUCHS, S., HAUX, R., ROSSLER, R., RUPPRECHT, B., SCHMELMER, V. and WIEGEL, S., 1994, Das Galenische Entwicklungs – System Heidelberg – Systematische Rezepturentwicklung, *Pharm. Ind.*, **56**, 641–647.

THOMAS, M., 1991, Expert systems in times of recession, *Manufacturing Intelligence*, **8**, 4–6.

TINSLEY, H., 1992, Expert systems in manufacturing, an overview, *Manufacturing Intelligence*, **9**, 7–9.

TURBAN, E., 1995, *Decision Support Systems and Expert Systems*, Englewood Cliffs, NJ: Prentice-Hall.

WOOD, M., 1991, Expert systems save formulation time, *Lab-Equipment Digest*, December, 17–19.

13

Future Prospects

13.1 Introduction

Intelligent software is a young technology by any standard. Although based on research dating back to the 1940s (neural networks), 1950s (expert systems) and 1960s (fuzzy logic), the technical feasibility and commercial availability has grown dramatically. In fact, intelligent systems should now be viewed as an important weapon in the armoury of senior management; the technology is mature and has proved its ability to generate real business benefits and competitive advantage. Applications in the domain of product formulation, although not commonplace, do exist, generating tangible benefits (Chapters 8, 9 and 10). Future prospects for the technology are discussed in this chapter under the headings Technology trends and Opportunities for product formulation.

13.2 Technology Trends

A view of the historical growth of computer capability over the past 40 years (Figure 13.1) shows the remarkable increase in computer speed as measured in floating point operations per second (FLOPS). Furthermore the cost of such capability as measured in dollars per million instructions per second (MIPS) is decreasing at the same logarithmic rate. The provision of more and more powerful personal computers at less and less cost has several consequences:

- The distinction between personal computers and workstations is blurring and much of the intelligent software originally generated on workstations is now being made available for personal computers.
- The increase in processing speed is decreasing the training time for neural networks, broadening their application.
- Very sophisticated software tools can now be supported by inexpensive computers.
- Lower overall cost of hardware makes justification of new applications of intelligent software easier.

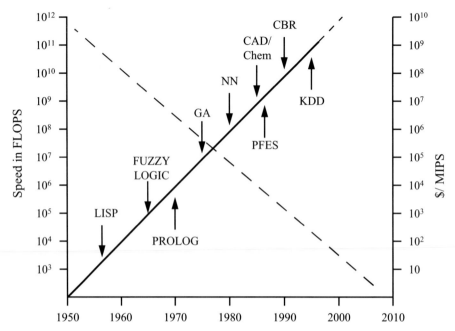

Figure 13.1 Speed and cost of computing since 1950 with selected highlights of intelligent software technology related to product formulation.
FLOPS, floating point operations per second; MIPS, million (10^6) instructions per second; GA, genetic algorithms; NN, neural networks; CAD/Chem, formulation modelling and optimisation (Chapter 6); PFES, product formulation expert system (Chapter 3); CBR, case-based reasoning; KDD, knowledge discovery in databases

All these will have an impact on the future research and development of intelligent software. Although symbolic (expert systems) and connectionist systems (neural networks, genetic algorithms) have both done very well in the complementary areas of classification and pattern recognition, in the future they will be increasingly involved in hybrid systems and integrated into conventional systems (databases, etc.). There are two major objectives to integration:

- enhancement of basic tools, e.g. expert systems can enhance neural computing, neural networks can enhance the knowledge acquisition of an expert system;
- enhancement of the capability of the application i.e. the tools compliment each other by performing subtasks at which the tool is best.

A very good example of software integration in the domain of product formulation is CAD/Chem (Chapter 6) containing (VerDuin, 1995):

- Neural network models to estimate properties for a given formulation.
- An expert system to run the models in consult mode.
- Fuzzy logic to specify ranking and preferences for product properties.
- Genetic algorithms for optimisation.

As well as being one of the first products to integrate all of these technologies it is also one of the first to focus on a specific application (VerDuin, 1995). Integration is also being seen in the construction of specialised tools for knowledge discovery in databases and data mining (Chapter 7).

Today the stand alone expert system is becoming rare; real world operational expert systems are increasingly being integrated with databases, management information systems, simulation and modelling programs. Expert systems integration with interactive multimedia and virtual reality will grow and knowledge-based simulation applications will be an important component in science and engineering. Combinations of neural networks and expert systems or neural networks and fuzzy logic will allow increasingly complex applications enhancing interest in, and acceptability of, neural networks. Areas not handled well with conventional computers will be appropriate for neural networks and connectionist systems run on parallel computers or optical computers; the latter, currently in the research phase, have the potential to perform at the speed of light.

Continued research in neural computing will minimise its limitations and expose further strengths in the approach. Collaboration between scientists in neurocomputing and neurobiology should lead to advances in the development of models to mimic human thinking and the processes that allow humans to make choices and reason.

The advances will be rapid because of national and international organisations and projects that are being initiated to address the opportunities of intelligent software. In Japan, following the success of the Fifth Generation Computer Project on knowledge-based systems (1982–1990), the Sixth Generation Computer Project on neural networks and fuzzy logic is now underway while the Seventh Generation Computer Project will focus on molecular computing (Steiner, 1991; Medsker and Liebowitz, 1994). In the USA, the 1990s have been designated the decade of the brain, resulting in increased work on neurocomputing.

The future looks bright for developments in intelligent software not only in its capability but also in its performance, the latter being due to the anticipated developments in hardware technology. The integration of complementary techniques will result in systems that will mimic human intelligence more closely providing opportunities for useful, practical and profitable applications.

13.3 Opportunities

Opportunities in the domain of product formulation are many: some are extensions of the applications already reviewed in Chapters 8, 9 and 10; some are just ideas, but all have the potential for changing working practices and delivering competitive edge.

13.3.1 Ab-initio *Formulation*

The concept of designing a formulation of a new chemical entity, *ab-initio*, knowing only its chemical formula, is one which has received much attention over recent years. Its success is dependent on the prediction of the properties of the chemical relevant to the formulation process and, with the recent introduction of modern modelling software packages in combination with formulation expert systems, the dream is very close to reality. In fact, elements of this approach can be clearly

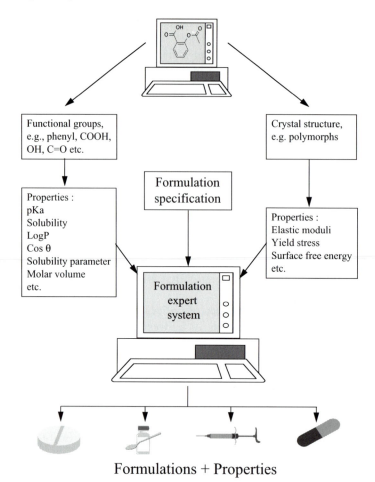

Formulations + Properties

Figure 13.2 Diagram of an integrated system for *ab-initio* formulation

seen in the expert system for formulating agrochemicals designed by personnel at Rohm and Haas (Hohne and Houghton, 1986). That system was interfaced to two FORTRAN programs, one a modelling program, the other a calculation program, to predict the solubility of the active ingredient in a range of solvents. A fully integrated system with more functionality is shown in Figure 13.2.

In such a system the user would enter the chemical structure of the molecule under examination plus the specification of the formulation (e.g. dose, concentration, type of formulation, etc.). An expert system would decide which modelling programs need to be accessed and what properties to predict. For example, if the formulation required the chemical to be in a powder form in a tablet, programs would be required to predict its crystal structure and possible polymorphs and calculate its mechanical properties relative to tabletting. Many such programs are now available (Table 13.1). Another expert system would then select the ingredients necessary for the formulation and the final formulation would be displayed. If, as in some cases, properties of formulations can be predicted, the expert system could produce a variety of formulations with predicted properties. This would allow the application of neural networks and genetic algorithms to optimise the formulation for specific desirable properties. If necessary, a recommended production process

Table 13.1 Some representative modelling/prediction programs and their suppliers

Program	Functionality	Supplier
pKalc 3.2	pKa	Compudrug Ltd, Hungary
Prolog P 5.1	LogP	Compudrug Ltd, Hungary
ClogP 2.0	LogP	BioByte Corp., USA
PrologD 2.0	LogD	Compudrug Ltd, Hungary
Cerius^2 Property prediction module	Elastic moduli	MSI, Cambridge
Cerius^2 Polymorph predictor	Crystal structure	MSI, Cambridge
Cerius^2 Morphology module	Crystal shape/surface energy	MSI, Cambridge
Cerius^2 Modelling environment	Van der Waals volume, Surface area, Molecular length, breadth, width, etc.	MSI, Cambridge

could also be included as an output. Such a system would allow decisions to be made regarding the cost effectiveness of the project and highlight possible problems, if any, at the outset of the project. The approach could also be used as part of a formulation screening process.

13.3.2 *Formulation Screening*

In those industries where formulations are required of an active chemical (e.g. pharmaceutical and agrochemical), combinatorial chemistry, which has the capacity to generate more candidate molecules in one year than used to be made in 30 years, is now being used extensively. It is an impossible task to prepare a sufficient amount of each molecule to prepare formulations especially if several types of formulation are to be considered. The concept of *ab-initio* formulation described above is one that lends itself to this problem. Formulations of various types could easily be screened for cost and possible problems at a very early stage, allowing decisions to be made regarding possible development and production.

13.3.3 *The Robot Formulator*

In many cases of product formulation, it is necessary to screen a series of trial formulations for chemical/physical stability since these properties are often very difficult to predict. Expert systems are very useful in this respect since as well as recommending an initial formulation they could also recommend a series of trial formulations with storage conditions to produce the optimum amount of stability data for a neural network/genetic algorithm to model and optimise. If such a concept was incorporated in a robotic system, it would be possible to screen a large number of formulations automatically with little human input. Robots and automated equipment are now present in many analytical laboratories and hence this concept of the robot formulator is not as far fetched as it would appear at first sight.

13.3.4 *Integrated Formulation/Process Design*

In the traditional product formulation design approach, a formulation is produced, tested and then the formulation/technology is transferred to the production department. If the product formulators are experienced and have knowledge of the production equipment, the formulation should have been designed such that it would have few problems, if any, on scale-up. This is not always the case: the formulator may have used small scale equipment very different from production plant; he may even have used materials difficult to manipulate on production scale. In this case the formulation would have to be revised incurring cost and resource penalties. In integrated formulation/process design the manufacturing impact of the formulation is considered at the outset. Changes can be made early in the design cycle where they will be easier and cheaper to implement. By viewing the formulation task in a broader context it is possible to improve manufacturing quality and decrease costs.

This integration requires more than an appropriate environment, it requires expertise on the interaction between product formulation and processing. This expertise is scarce especially if processing is carried out at a different location from where the formulation is developed. Expert systems have already been shown to be applicable for product formulation and some do already have links to the processing equipment (see WOOLY for wool dyeing and TEXPERTO for textile finishing, Chapter 8). The strengthening of this link by the incorporation of more knowledge of the processing equipment to be used, possibly with modelling and simulation, should provide the environment necessary to optimise across design, materials and processing from the outset of the project.

It should be emphasised that this approach is different from the formulation modelling and optimisation approach used in CAD/Chem (Chapter 6). In the CAD/Chem approach it is assumed that the experimental data relating formulation and processing are available. In the integrated formulation/process design approach the formulation produced should have all the attributes necessary for it to be manufactured successfully.

The potential benefits of such an approach are obvious: quality products faster at lower cost and with more efficient processing.

13.3.5 *Integrated Formulation Management*

For specialty chemical companies in business to supply bespoke formulations of their products to meet customer demands, the creation of an integrated formulation management system could certainly lead to increased competitive edge. A relatively simple system integrating administration, formulation, production and testing tasks within a generic, research and application development is shown in Figure 13.3. It is based on a local area network (LAN) of personal computers and consists of four main parts:

- A formulation selection system to develop formulations to meet customer requirements. As well as containing a formulation expert system, it has links to databases on past formulations, ingredients and properties (results from testing procedures).

- A production management expert system to which are connected various automated processing equipment via real-time, on-line, knowledge-based systems

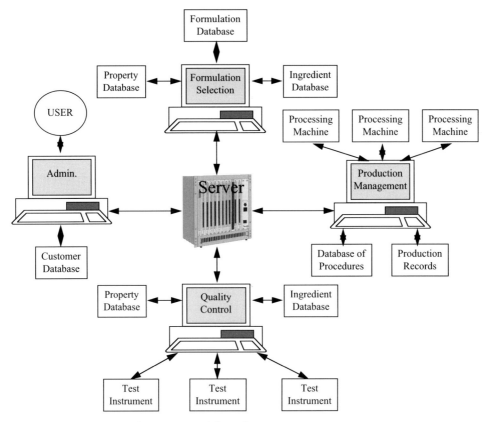

Figure 13.3 Diagram of an integrated formulation management system

similar to those described by Taunton (1992). The system also has links to databases of procedures and production records.

- A testing and quality control expert system connected to various testing instruments as well as being linked to databases on test methods and standards.
- An administration system through which the user accesses all the information including a customer database.

With such a system it will be possible to handle a large number of queries from customers, developing bespoke quality formulations with the correct properties and manufactured to time. It is inevitable that such a system would deliver tangible benefits in terms of quality of service, increased response, decreased costs and increased revenue and profitability (Figure 11.7). In fact, less developed systems without embedded expert systems have proved feasible and delivered benefits (Visser, 1992). Such a system would be able to generate a large amount of quality data suitable for modelling using neural networks or data mining.

13.3.6 *Experience Provision*

In the real world, product formulation is more of a task born of experience than one born of science and technology. For instance, despite all the progress made over the past three decades in understanding the principles of powder compaction, pharmaceutical tablet formulation is still regarded by some more as an art than a science. Of course, an understanding of the basic principles is essential and is generally taught in university courses. However, no amount of formal education can take the place of experience in equipping the tablet formulator to make the correct decisions.

Essentially experience is knowledge acquired over time working on real projects under the watchful eye of supervisors, peers, mentors and, possibly, customers; making mistakes and having them corrected. In fact, it is generally accepted that more is learnt from failures than from successes. Hence experience is nothing unless there is real hands-on work with real materials, costing real money, in real time and with real people. The question is how this can be accomplished in an environment like product formulation that is being constrained in resources and time in a general culture of low tolerance of failure. One method is the use of intelligent software systems. At the lowest level this could be the adoption of interactive expert systems for product development where the novice formulator could formulate real drugs to real specifications in real time. Product formulation expert systems now exist for a wide range of formulation types (Chapter 8). In fact, several uses of this technology have reported a benefit in the training of novice formulators (Chapter 11). However, in order to make such systems more useful other features need to be considered:

- It is essential that all expert systems include a logical and comprehensive explanation of their reasoning in a language understandable to the novice.

- An essential element of gaining experience is the inclusion of all human senses (sight, hearing, touch, smell, taste) in describing an event. For instance, if a tablet formulation contains insufficient lubricant its performance on a tablet machine will change over time. The noise generated by the machine might change as the tablets become either difficult to eject or even become jammed in the die. In such an event it is essential to include video images and sound alongside the expert system.

A concept, not beyond the realms of possibility, is that of using virtual reality whereby a formulator, sat at a computer, could perform all the tasks from formulation to processing using real-time expert systems to advise, correct mistakes if necessary, and provide explanations for all events. All senses, possibly with the exception of smell, could be included and failure could be tolerated as it would not have any concrete effect. Thus experience could be gained comparable with that obtained by conventional means. This is in essence a formulation development simulator.

13.3.7 *The Reasoning Notebook*

The examples of applications of expert systems discussed in Chapters 8 and 9 have established convincingly that systems which correspond behaviourally to a formulator at a given time can be easily constructed. However, in an environment where the formulator's behaviour has to adapt to meet changes in requirements and understanding, rule-based expert systems have problems and cannot encompass adequately the activity of the formulator. This problem has, to some extent, been addressed by case-based reasoning. This type of reasoning is more adaptive than rule-based and, as has been proven, is intrinsically a learning methodology (Chapter 4).

It is inevitable that case-based reasoning will be applied extensively to product formulation in the future. In fact, several prototype applications in pharmaceutical formulation are currently being developed and evaluated. If, as expected, the technology can deliver the benefits claimed for it and is relatively easy to apply, the problem of adaptation to changes in formulation behaviour can be addressed.

A concept, not beyond the realms of possibility, is the reasoning notebook. In this a formulator when starting a new project would enter each new formulation, as it is conceived, into a computer in a similar fashion to using a notebook. This would be seen as a case by case-based reasoning shell that would automatically index each formulation. Such a system would then be able to assist the formulator in generating new formulations and, as the case-base becomes larger, it will learn and become more efficient. If the project was then abandoned for some reason or other, all the data could be archived. Each new project would be treated as a new case-base. Such a concept is compatible with the provision of corporate memory.

13.3.8 *Corporate Memory*

A vital asset of organisations is the knowledge and experience of their employees. There are two types of corporate knowledge – product specific and skill specific knowledge – and both are required for effective performance. Staff turnover and reorganisation through, for example, a merger, can result in loss of corporate memory leading, in some cases, to the reinvention of the wheel. When case-based systems are augmented by the experiences of those who use them, they become a corporate memory for the organisation that is using them. Probably the best illustration to date is the system known as CLAVIER designed by personnel at Lockheed in Palo Alto, California for the configuration of autoclave loads (Keen, 1993, and described in Chapter 4). Case-based reasoning has recently been used as part of an experience – sharing architecture in the NEC Corporation in Japan (Kitano and Shimazu, 1996).

13.4 **Conclusion**

As can be seen, rapid developments in intelligent software technology have created an environment in which there are many opportunities for applications in the domain of product formulation. In an era of escalating competition and an increasing skills shortage among product formulators, the industrial winners will be those companies that can seize and exploit this technology as a strategic weapon. The challenge is to translate opportunity into action and the ideas presented in this chapter are intended to provide a perspective that may be useful in identifying new applications.

References

HOHNE, B.A. and HOUGHTON, R.D., 1986, An expert system for the formulation of agricultural chemicals, in PIERCE, T.H. and HOHNE, B.A. (eds.), *Artificial Intelligence Applications in Chemistry*, ACS Symposium series 306, pp. 87–97, Chicago: American Chemical Society.

KITANO, H. and SHIMAZU, H., 1996, The experience-sharing architecture: a case study in corporate wide case-based software quality control, in LEAKE, D.B. (ed.), *Cased-Based Reasoning, Experiences, Lessons and Future Directions*, pp. 235–268, Menlo Park, CA: AAAI Press.

KEEN, M.J.R., 1993, Successful applications of case-based reasoning, *Manufacturing Intelligence*, **14**, 10–12.

MEDSKER, L. and LIEBOWITZ, J., 1994, *Design and Development of Expert Systems and Neural Networks*, New York: Macmillan.

STEINER, J., 1991, Overview of manufacturing intelligence in Japan, *Manufacturing Intelligence*, **8**, 15–17.

TAUNTON, C., 1992, G2 – a real-time expert system tool for integrated on line manufacturing applications, *Manufacturing Intelligence*, **12**, 8–11.

VERDUIN, W.H., 1995, *Better Products Faster*, New York: Irwin.

Visser, G.W., 1992, Integrated computerised system for formulations, mixing and testing of materials, *Rubber World*, **205** (5), 20–28.

An Example Formulation Expert System

In this appendix a series of screen images has been used to illustrate the operation of a typical formulation expert system. The system for formulating tablets uses PFES from Logica (Chapter 3) and is similar to that described in Chapter 9.

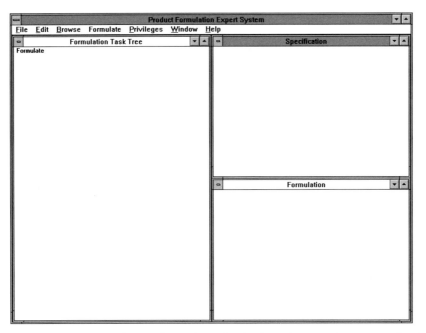

Figure A1.1 The user interface with windows for the formulation task tree, specification and formulation. Tasks are deployed in various formats: highlighted text – current task; italics – completed tasks; standard text – future tasks. Selection of the 'Formulate' option causes the system to start

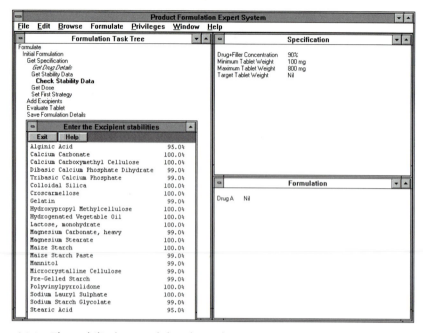

Figure A1.2 The stability/compatibility data relevant to Drug A (the selected drug). The values are the percentage of the drug remaining after mixtures of the drug and excipient have been stored under specified conditions of temperature and humidity. It is possible to amend the data at this stage but the amendments are deleted on shutdown and are not stored in the database which is password protected. It can be seen that the specification window already contains a series of generic, high-level targets for the tablet formulation

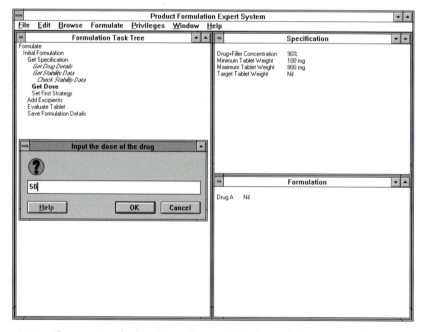

Figure A1.3 The user is asked to input the required dose of the drug (in this case 50 mg)

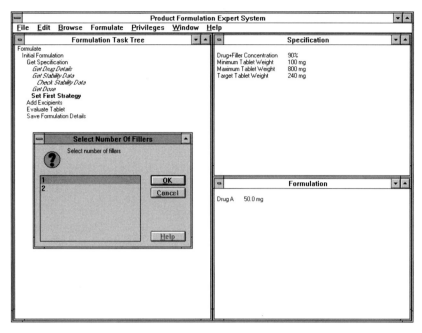

Figure A1.4 The user is asked to input the number of fillers required (1 in this case). It can be seen that the specification window now contains a target tablet weight calculated using a formula determined from an extensive study of previous formulations

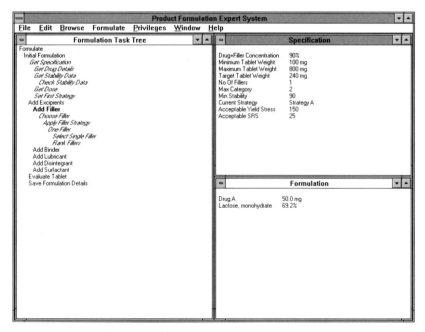

Figure A1.5 The specification window now contains a series of targets for the final tablet specified in terms of the minimum acceptable excipient stability/compatibility and acceptable compression properties. The system has selected lactose monohydrate at a level of 69.2% as the filler satisfying these criteria

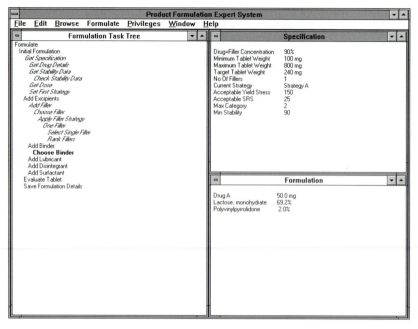

Figure A1.6   The system has selected polyvinylpyrrolidone at a level of 2.0% as the binder satisfying the target specification and excipient selection criteria

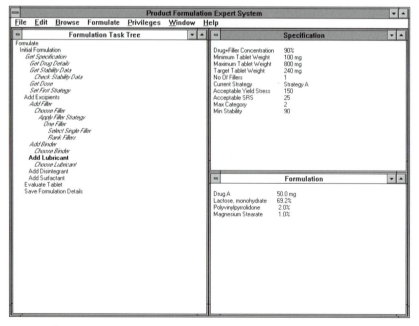

Figure A1.7   The system has selected magnesium stearate at a level of 1.0% as the lubricant satisfying the target specification excipient selection criteria

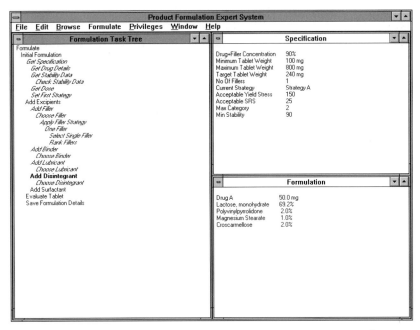

Figure A1.8 The system has selected croscarmellose at a level of 2.0% as the disintegrant satisfying the target specification and excipient selection criteria

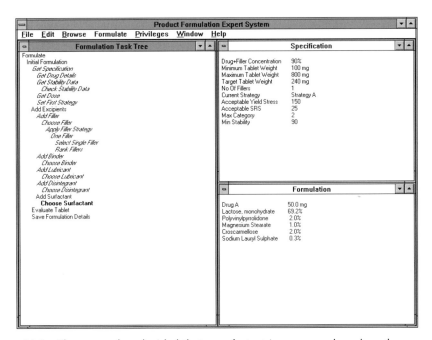

Figure A1.9 The system has decided that a surfactant is necessary based on the properties of the selected drug and has selected sodium lauryl sulphate at a level of 0.3% as the surfactant satisfying the target specification

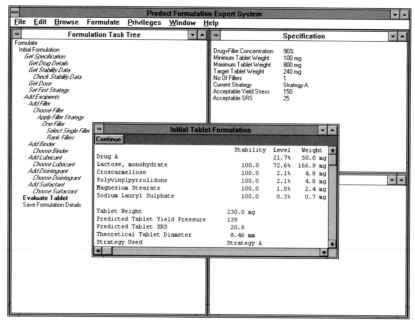

Figure A1.10   The recommended tablet formulation expressed both as a weight percentage and as mg/tablet is displayed together with predictions of its compression properties. A recommended tablet diameter is included for reference

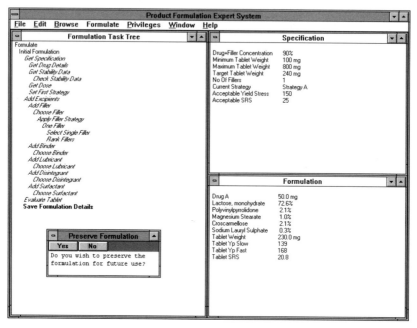

Figure A1.11   An option is provided to preserve the formulation and store it in a database for future reference or delete it

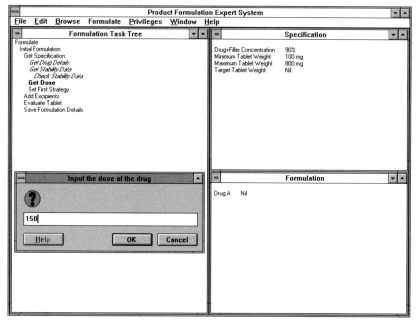

Figure A1.12   In order to initiate the formulation of a tablet with a different dose of drug, the 'get dose' task is selected and the user asked to input the new dose (in this case 150 mg)

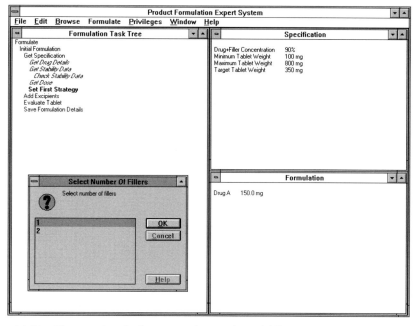

Figure A1.13   The user is asked to input the number of fillers required (1 in this case). It can be seen that the target tablet weight is now 350 mg (cf. 240 mg for the 50 mg dose)

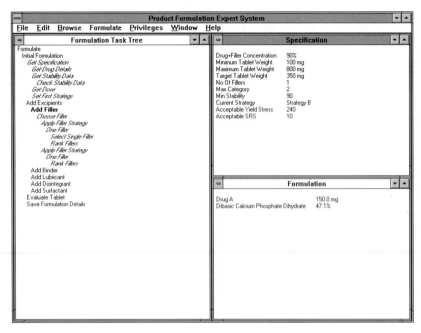

Figure A1.14 The system has selected dibasic calcium phosphate dihydrate at a level of 47.1%, satisfying the new specification for the 150 mg dose

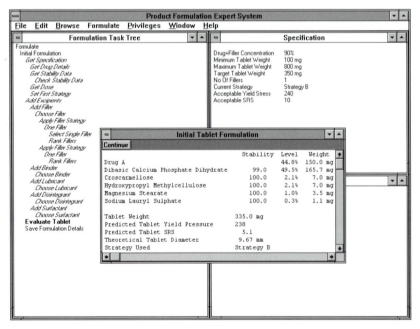

Figure A1.15 The recommended tablet formulation for the 150 mg dose is displayed. A comparison with that for the 50 mg dose (Figure A1.10) shows differences in both the filler and binder chosen

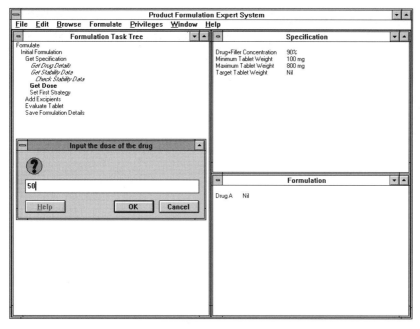

Figure A1.16 In order to initiate the formulation of a tablet with two fillers, the 'get dose' task is selected and the user asked to input the dose of the drug required (in this case 50 mg)

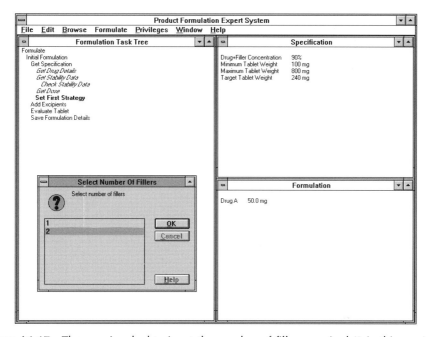

Figure A1.17 The user is asked to input the number of fillers required (2 in this case)

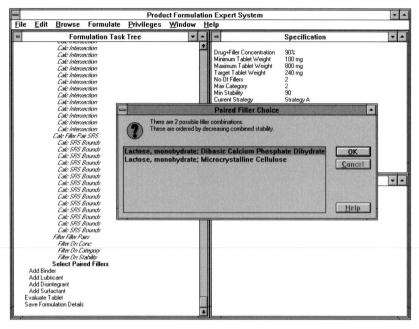

Figure A1.18   The system searches its database for possible further combinations satisfying the tablet specification and has suggested two possible combinations ordered by decreasing stability/compatibility. The user is then asked to select one – in this case the most highly recommended one

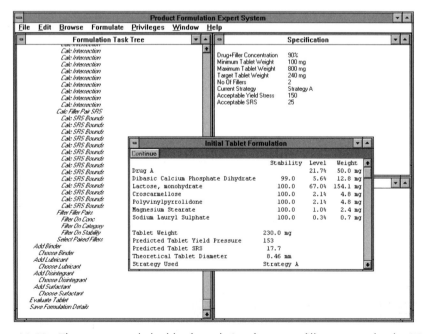

Figure A1.19   The recommended tablet formulation for a two filler strategy for the 50 mg dose is displayed

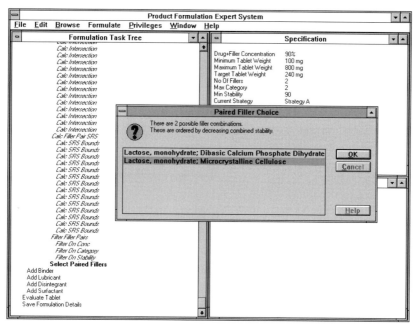

Figure A1.20   If the user selects the second recommended filler combination in preference then see Figure A1.21

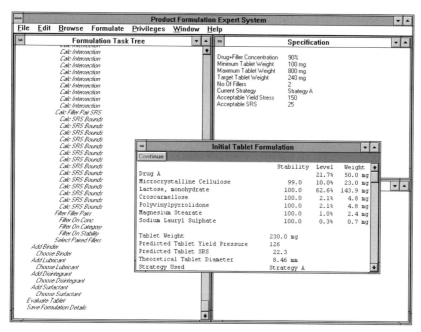

Figure A1.21   A new tablet formulation is displayed. It can be seen that this formulation has very similar compression properties to that shown in Figure A1.19

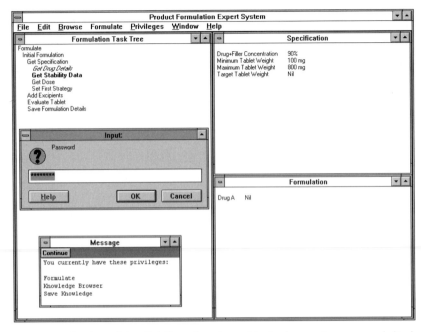

Figure A1.22 Selection of the 'Privileges' option with the input of a password displays the privileges of the user. In this case the user is not allowed to alter higher level options e.g. edit the knowledge base

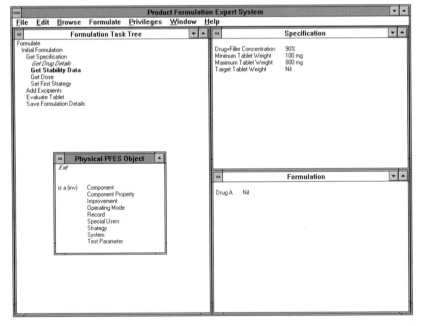

Figure A1.23 Selection of the 'Browse' option allows the user to browse the knowledge base. By selecting the Component option the user is able to browse all knowledge pertaining to the components of the formulation

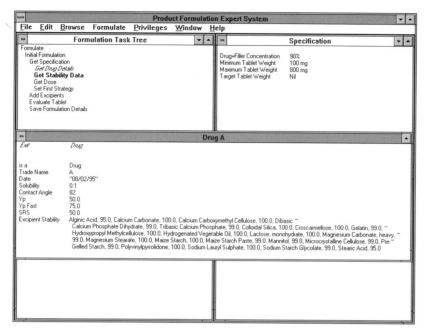

Figure A1.24 This shows the data for Drug A including its solubility (mg ml⁻¹), contact angle with water, compression properties and excipient stability/compatibility

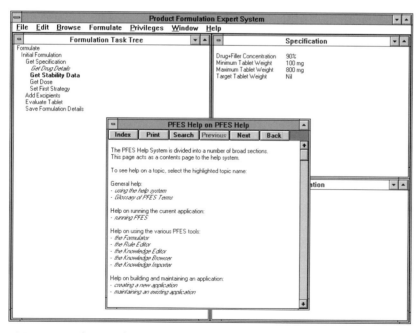

Figure A1.25 By selecting the 'Help' option the user is able to access help messages both for operating the system and information on the system

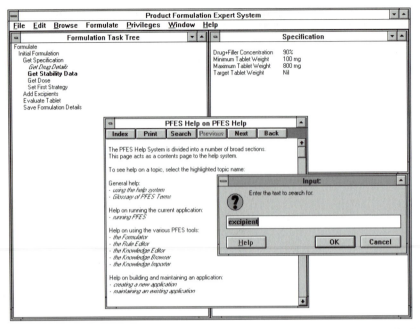

Figure A1.26   A search routine has been included and the user is asked to specify the text to search for (in this case excipient)

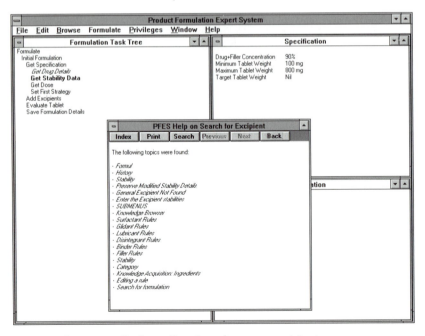

Figure A1.27   The system displays all topics relevant to excipients

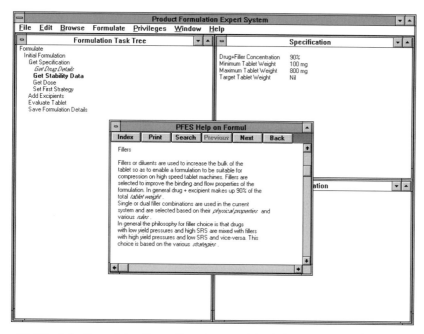

Figure A1.28 Selection of the 'Formul' option provides information on fillers relevant to the formulation process

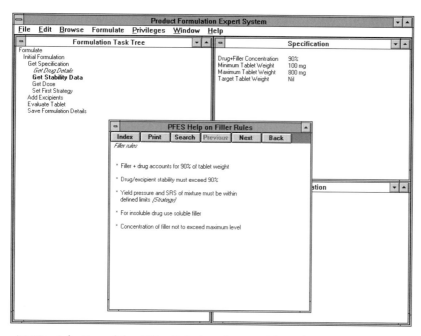

Figure A1.29 Selection of the 'Filler Rules' option provides information on the rules used to select filler

APPENDIX 2

An Example Fault Diagnosis Expert System

In this appendix a series of screen images has been used to illustrate the operation of a typical fault diagnosis expert system. The system for the identification and solution of defects on film coated tablets uses 1st Class from Trinzic Corp. and is similar to that described in Chapter 9. It uses the decision tree shown in Figure 4.2 to identify the defect.

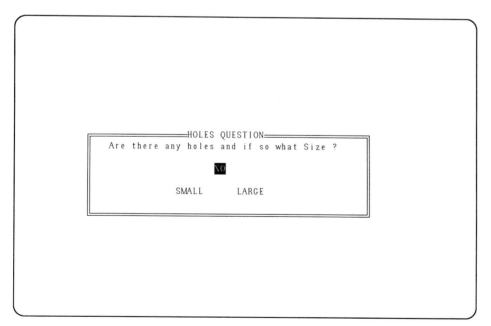

Figure A2.1 The first question regarding the presence of holes and of what size. An answer in the negative causes the system to proceed to another question

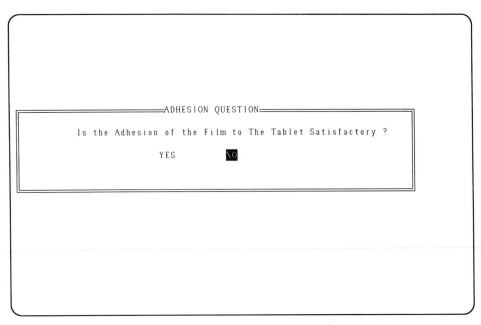

Figure A2.2   The second question regarding the adhesion of the film to the tablet. An answer in the negative causes the system to proceed to another question

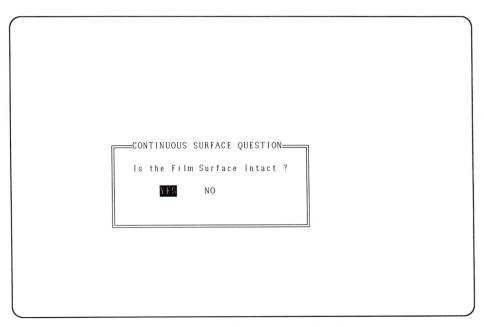

Figure A2.3   The third question regarding the continuity of the film. An answer in the affirmative causes the system to proceed to another question

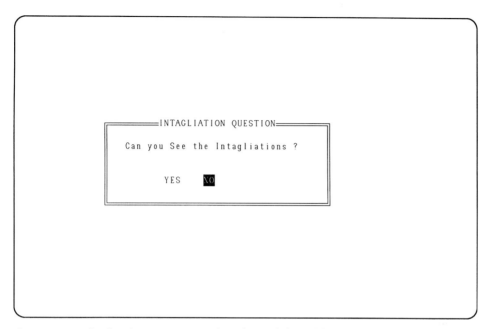

Figure A2.4 The fourth question regarding the visibility of the intagliations (lettering or design in relief on the tablet). An answer in the negative results in a diagnosis

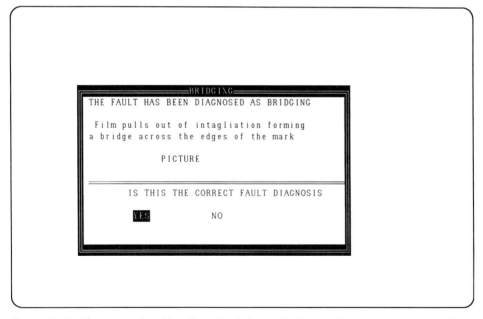

Figure A2.5 The system has identified the defect as bridging of the intagliations, briefly describes it and presents a picture if required. The user is then asked to confirm the diagnosis. An answer in the affirmative causes the system to proceed to the second stage

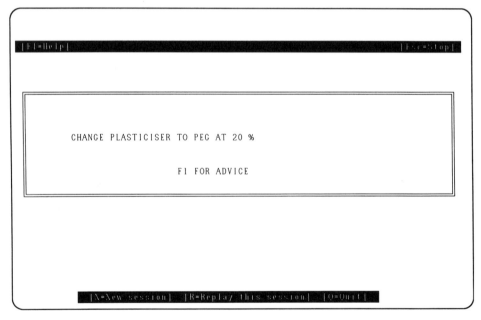

```
═══════════════COMPONENT QUESTION BRIDGING═══════════════
              PLEASE ENTER THE FOLLOWING DATA

AIR INLET TEMP  :  60  °C

EXHAUST TEMP    :  35  °C

SPRAY RATE      :  50  ml/MIN

SOLUTION CONC   :  7.5  %

      PLASTICISER GLYCEROL   PLASTICISER CONC 20

          SELECT LIST              SELECT LIST
      PEG  GLYCEROL      10      20      30
      PG   NONE

      INCIDENCE:HIGH     CHANGE FORMULATION:YES
      LOW                               YES
      HIGH                              NO


              PRESS TO CONTINUE
```

Figure A2.6   The user is asked to enter the relevant processing conditions and formulation details regarding the defect

```
[F1=Help]                                      [Esc=Stop]



 ┌──────────────────────────────────────────────────────┐
 │                                                        │
 │         CHANGE PLASTICISER TO PEG AT 20 %              │
 │                                                        │
 │              F1 FOR ADVICE                             │
 │                                                        │
 └──────────────────────────────────────────────────────┘



        [N=New session]  [R=Replay this session]  [Q=Quit]
```

Figure A2.7   The system presents a solution to the problem: in this case changing the plasticiser but maintaining its concentration

```
══════════════════════════════BRIDGING NOTES══════════════════════════

                  Generally caused by High Internal Stresses.
      Bridging can be overcome by changing the geometry of the intagliations,
          wide/deep intagliations being better than narrow/shallow ones.

                        Bridging is often associated with
                                   SPLITTING
                                      and
                                    CRACKING

                True Bridging can be distinguished from INFILLING
                  as the Bridge can be easily deformed and pushed back into
                      the intagliation by means of a rounded pin-head

                        PICTURE 1          PICTURE 2

                                  REFERENCES
```

Figure A2.8   Selection of the Help routine displays notes regarding the defect. Hypertext links can be used to access the other defects mentioned and also pictures and references

```
══════════════════════════════BRIDGING PAPERS═════════════════════════

        THE EFFECT OF FILM THICKNESS ON THE INCIDENCE OF THE
    DEFECT BRIDGING OF THE INTAGLIATIONS ON FILM COATED TABLETS

          R.C.ROWE S.F.FORSE J. PHARM PHARMACOL 1980 32 647-648


                        ─────────────────


        THE EFFECT OF PLASTICISER TYPE AND CONCENTRATION ON THE INCIDENCE
          OF BRIDGING OF INTAGLIATIONS OF FILM COATED TABLETS

          R.C.ROWE S.F.FORSE J. PHARM PHARMACOL 1981 33 174-175


                        ─────────────────


        THE EFFECT OF INTAGLIATION SHAPE ON THE INCIDENCE OF BRIDGING
                      ON FILM COATED TABLETS

          R.C.ROWE S.F.FORSE J. PHARM PHARMACOL 1981 33 423-426


                        ─────────────────                      ↓PgDn
```

Figure A2.9   Selection of 'References' causes the system to display all references relative to the defect

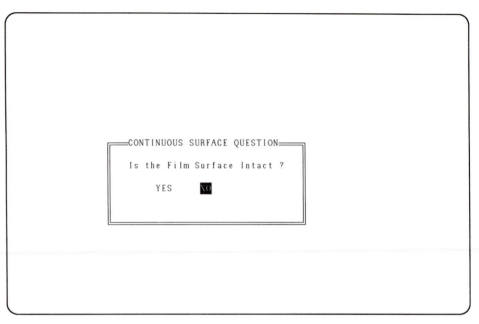

Figure A2.10 If the user had answered the third question regarding the continuity of the film (Figure A2.3) in the negative, the system reacts in a different way

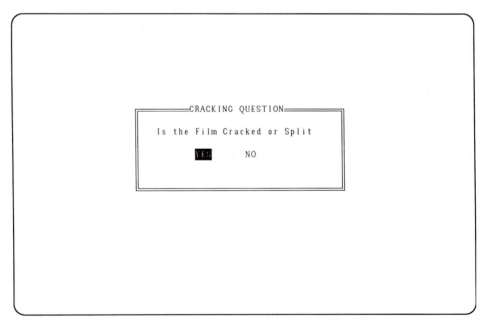

Figure A2.11 The new fourth question (cf. Figure A2.4) regarding the presence of cracks in the film. An answer in the affirmative results in a diagnosis

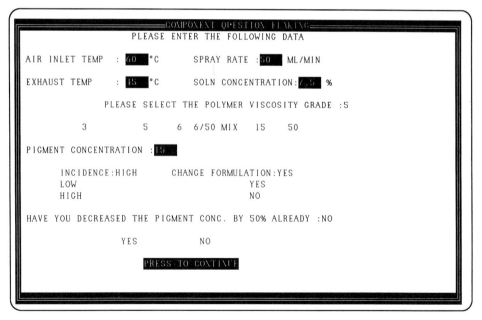

```
                      ═FLAKING═
┌──────────────────────────────────────────────┐
│                                                │
│  THE FAULT HAS BEEN DIAGNOSED AS FLAKING       │
│                                                │
│    Film flakes off exposing the                │
│        tablet surface                          │
│                                                │
│                                                │
│         PICTURE                                │
│                                                │
├────────────────────────────────────────────────┤
│                                                │
│     IS THIS THE CORRECT FAULT DIAGNOSIS        │
│                                                │
│     YES            NO                          │
│                                                │
└──────────────────────────────────────────────┘
```

Figure A2.12 The system has identified the defect as flaking, briefly describes it and presents a picture if required. As before, if the user confirms the diagnosis the system proceeds to the second stage

```
                  ═COMPONENT QUESTION FLAKING═
              PLEASE ENTER THE FOLLOWING DATA

AIR INLET TEMP   : 60  °C      SPRAY RATE : 50  ML/MIN

EXHAUST TEMP     : 45  °C      SOLN CONCENTRATION: 7.5  %

          PLEASE SELECT THE POLYMER VISCOSITY GRADE :5

      3          5     6  6/50 MIX   15    50

PIGMENT CONCENTRATION : 15

     INCIDENCE:HIGH       CHANGE FORMULATION:YES
     LOW                             YES
     HIGH                            NO

HAVE YOU DECREASED THE PIGMENT CONC. BY 50% ALREADY :NO

          YES              NO

              PRESS TO CONTINUE
```

Figure A2.13 Again the user is asked to enter all relevant process and formulation details. It should be noted that this time the questions are different since they are only relevant to the new defect

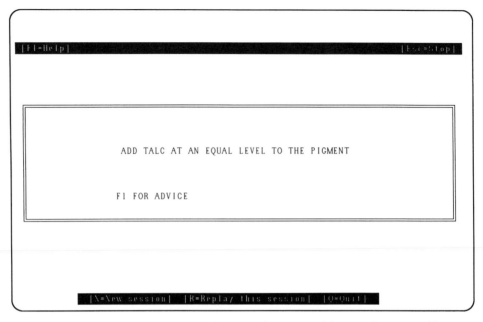

Figure A2.14 The system presents a solution to the new problem: in this case adding a quantity of talc equal to the quantity of pigment already in the formulation

Glossary

The following glossary is intended to provide a brief definition of some of the terms used in this book that relate to intelligent software technology only. It does not incorporate terminology specific to the formulation domain or any of the applications described.

adaptive A system that adapts or modifies its behaviour to suit changing circumstances.

algorithm A procedure, often a set of equations, for solving a problem.

artificial intelligence A field of computer science that is concerned with symbolic reasoning and problem solving in an attempt to reproduce human intelligence.

artificial neural network Model systems for computation based on nerves and their behaviour.

attribute A characteristic of an object.

auto-associative neural networks A special form of the multi-layer perceptron consisting of two MLP networks connected back to back with a common middle layer.

back-propagation A technique for computing the required adjustment to the weights of the neurons during supervised training of a neural network.

backward chaining A method of reasoning starting with a hypothesis and finding data to prove or disprove it.

Bayesian probability The probability of a particular event computed using Bayes theorem allowing the revision of existing probability based on new information.

breadth-first search A routine by which a search is initiated at a specific level on each branch in turn before moving to a different level.

case-based reasoning (CBR) A methodology in which old solutions to a problem are adapted to meet new demands.

causal network Similar to a semantic network but where the links are used to express causation.

conjugate gradient algorithm A special form of line search algorithm used for computing the required adjustments to the weights of the neurons during supervised training of neural networks.

conventional languages Standard computing languages such as FORTRAN, PASCAL or C.

data mining The application of algorithms for extracting patterns and useful knowledge from data.

decision support system (DSS) A computer based information system that combines models and data in an attempt to solve non-structural problems.

decision table A way of representing knowledge in a tabular form.

decision tree A way of representing knowledge in the form of a tree with branches and leaf nodes.

declarative knowledge A descriptive representation of the facts pertaining to a domain.

defuzzification A process by which a fuzzy output is combined with an output membership function to produce a precise output.

depth-first search A routine by which a search is initiated downward along a given branch until a solution or dead end is reached. In the latter the process backtracks to the first alternative branch and tries again.

desirability function A description of the relative desirability of different parameter values across the allowable range of that parameter. Used in optimisation routines.

domain knowledge Knowledge and expertise about a particular field.

dynamic analysis The evaluation of the functionality of a system which involves the execution of the system.

environment Development systems that support several different ways of representing knowledge and handling inference.

epoch One complete pass through the training set in a neural network.

expert system A computer program that either recommends or makes decisions for people based on the knowledge gathered from experts in the field.

explicit knowledge Knowledge the domain expert is conscious of having and is able to articulate.

feed-forward network A generic term for a neural network in which the signals are passed in the forward direction only.

flexible tolerance method (FTM) A method of optimisation using the principles of hill-climbing to find the maximum or minimum on a surface.

forward chaining A method of reasoning from data to form a hypothesis.

frame A template for holding clusters of related knowledge about a particular object.

functional link neural (FLN) networks A special form of the multi-layer perceptron in which the neurons in both the input and hidden layers are enhanced using linear or trigonometric functions.

fuzzification A process by which a real-time input is combined with information on input membership functions to produce fuzzy inputs.

fuzzy logic A method of reasoning that can cope with uncertain or partial information.

fuzzy sets A set of elements without a crisp or precise boundary.

Gaussian functional link network (GFLN) A special form of the radial basis function network in which the input neurons contain an additional statistical transformation.

generalisation The ability of a neural network to produce sensible outputs when presented with data that were not used to train it.

genetic algorithm An optimisation technique based on the evolutionary process by which biological systems self-organise and adapt.

guided evolutionary simulated annealing (GESA) A method of optimisation which combines the principles of both genetic algorithms and simulated annealing.

heuristics Rules of thumb or informal judgemental knowledge of a domain.

hidden layer Middle layer of neurons in a neural network.

hierarchy A structure arranged in a branching form whereby each level denotes the relative importance of the objects(s) in that level.

hypertext An approach for handling text by allowing the user to undertake jumps from a given topic to any other related topic.

ID3 A specific algorithm used to generate a decision tree.

inference engine That part of an expert system that simulates the problem solving process.

inheritance A process by which one object takes on or is assigned the characteristics of another object higher up the hierarchy.

input layer Layer of neurons in a neural network representing the input data.

interface That part of the computer system that interacts with the user.

knowledge acquisition The extraction of knowledge derived from various sources.

knowledge base That part of an expert system where all knowledge and expertise concerning the problem domain is stored.

knowledge-based information system (KBIS) See expert system.

knowledge discovery in databases (KDD) The non-trivial process of identifying valid, novel, potentially useful and understandable patterns in data.

knowledge drift The change in knowledge that occurs slowly with time.

knowledge engineer A specialist responsible for the technical side of developing an expert system.

knowledge engineering The structuring of knowledge obtained from domain experts and other sources such that it can be integrated into a computer and used by non-experts.

knowledge refinement The correction of errors in the rule-base of an expert system triggered when test cases are wrongly solved.

knowledge representation The formalism of representing facts and rules about a domain in a computer.

Kohonen networks A self-organising map consisting of a single layer of neurons.

leaf node Node in a search tree with no successions designating the end of the search.

learning vector quantisation (LVQ) networks A special form of the multi-layer perceptron providing discrete rather than continuous outputs.

line search algorithms A series of algorithms used for computing the required adjustments to the weights of the neurons during supervised training of a neural network.

membership function A characteristic function of each element within a fuzzy set.

metaknowledge Knowledge about how a system operates or reasons – knowledge about knowledge.

multi-layer perceptron (MLP) network A form of neural network consisting of identical neurons arranged in interconnected layers.

natural language processing (NLP) A technology by which a user is able to carry on a conversation with a computer based system.

neural computing A technology that attempts to mimic the processing capabilities of the human brain.

neural network A technology that attempts to mimic the processing capabilities of the human brain using simple logic processing units (neurons) organised in specific arrangements (neural network architecture).

neural network architecture The method by which the neurons are organised.

neuron The fundamental logic processing unit of the neural network.

object A fragment of knowledge encompassing everything to do with an idea or item. Objects may be physical or conceptual.

output layer Layer of neurons in a neural network representing the output data.

overtraining This is where training has been carried on to a point where the neural network starts to learn the noise in the training examples resulting in poor generalisation.

procedural knowledge A detailed set of instructions about courses of action.

production rule A conditional statement that specifies an action or actions to be taken under a certain set of conditions.

prototyping A strategy whereby a portion of a system is constructed in a short time, tested and refined over several iterations.

radial basis function (RBF) network A form of neural network in which the neurons in the hidden layer contain statistical transformations.

Rapson–Newton method A method of optimisation using defined rules.

recurrent neural network A form of neural network in which the output not only depends on the input but also on the previous inputs and values of the internal activations in the network.

root node The initial state node of a search tree.

rule induction A methodology that automatically extracts information in the form of a set of rules or a decision tree from a set of examples.

schema A data structure, a pattern matching template.

schema theorem A theorem that describes the rate that schema proliferate.

semantic network A graphical depiction of the relationships (links) between objects (nodes).

shell A computer program capable of being an expert system when loaded with the relevant knowledge.

simulated annealing A method of optimisation based on the physical principles underlying the controlled cooling of metals and glasses. The value of the objective function to be minimised is analogous to the energy in a thermodynamic system.

slot A sub-element of a frame.

software kernel An expert system shell with specific knowledge representative structures capable of being an application when loaded with the relevant knowledge.

Spearman rank coefficient An indication of the degree of correlation between two variables.

special purpose languages Special computing languages such as LISP and PROLOG developed for artificial intelligence applications.

spreadsheet A template for holding information in columns and rows.

static analysis A manual or automatic examination of the information/data contained in a system which does not involve the execution of the system.

stochastic algorithm An algorithm that relies on random elements in parts of its operation.

supervised training A process by which a neural network is presented with a series of matching input and output examples and the weights of the neurons are adjusted such that the output for a specific input is the same or close to the desired output.

symbolic processing The use of symbols combined with rules to process information and to solve problems.

tacit knowledge Knowledge the domain expert is not conscious of having but does exist as proved by the expert's known capability of solving problems.

task A well defined activity.

training The process whereby the weights of the neurons in a neural network are varied in order to achieve optimal performance.

transformation (activation) function A mathematical function to model the output level of a neuron to a level between zero and one.

Turing testing A method of validating an expert system by comparing the results of the expert system with those from a human expert on the same set of test cases.

uncertainty The unreliability or incompleteness of the information/knowledge in an expert system.

unsupervised training A process by which a neural network is presented with input data only and the weights of the neurons are adjusted such that similar inputs consistently result in the same output.

validation A method of substantiating whether a system has attained an adequate level of performance with an acceptable level of accuracy and reliability.

verification A method of substantiating whether a system correctly implements its specification.

virtual reality A three-dimensional interactive technology providing the user with a feeling of being present in the real world.

weights The values of the strength of the connections in a neural network.

workstation A class of computers exceeding the capability of the personal computer characterised by an emphasis on computational power.

APPENDIX 4

Acronyms

The following acronyms are used in this book:

AI	artificial intelligence
ANOVA	analysis of variance
CAD	computer aided design
CBR	case-based reasoning
DOS	disk operating system
DSS	decision support system
DTI	Department of Trade and Industry
FL	fuzzy logic
FLN	functional link neural (network)
FLOPS	floating point operations per second
FTM	flexible tolerance method
GA	genetic algorithm
GESA	guided evolutionary simulated annealing
GFLN	Gaussian functional link network
HPLC	high performance liquid chromatography
KBIS	knowledge-based information systems
KDD	knowledge discovery in databases
LAN	local area network
LVQ	learning vector quantisation (network)
MB	megabyte
MIPS	million (10^6) instructions per second
MLP	multi-layer perceptron
NLP	natural language processing

NN	neural network
PC	personal computer
PFES	Product Formulation Expert System
PVC	polvinyl chloride
PVP	polyvinyl pyrrolidone
RAM	random access memory
RBF	radial basis function (network)
RI	rule induction

Biographical Notes

Raymond C. Rowe Ray Rowe is a Company Research Associate at Zeneca Pharmaceuticals, UK. He supervises a team engaged in research and problem solving in all areas of physical sciences (including colloid science, powder technology and knowledge engineering) involved in the formulation of medicines. He has been with Zeneca Pharmaceuticals (formally ICI Pharmaceuticals) since 1973 having received his BPharm from the University of Nottingham in 1969 and his PhD from the University of Manchester in 1973.

His research interests lie in the area of polymer coating, powder technology including compaction and granulation, the structural characterisation of complex colloid systems and more recently, applications of knowledge engineering in formulation and analysis. He has published over 300 research papers and reviews including eight patents. In 1992 he was designated Fellow of the Royal Pharmaceutical Society for distinction in the Science of Pharmacy and in 1993 he was awarded a DSc from the University of Manchester. He is also a Fellow of the Royal Society of Chemistry and a Member of the Institute of Physics.

He has been an adjunct professor at the University of Illinois at Chicago and a visiting professor of the Universities of Strathclyde (Scotland) and at Santiago de Compestela (Spain). He is currently a visiting professor at the University of Bradford.

Ronald J. Roberts Ron Roberts is a Formulation Scientist at Zeneca Pharmaceuticals, UK and is currently responsible for the formulation development of new chemical entities. He has been with Zeneca Pharmaceuticals (formerly ICI Pharmaceuticals) since 1973, receiving his BSc in Chemistry from the Stockport College of Science and Technology in 1980 and PhD in Pharmaceutical Technology from the University of Bradford in 1992.

His research interests lie in the area of powder technology including comminution, compaction and the mechanical properties of pharmaceutical materials. He has published over 50 research papers and is currently a reviewer in these areas for a number of scientific journals.

Paul Bentley   Paul Bentley is a Principal Consultant with Logica UK Ltd. He has worked in the field of expert systems since 1988 and has managed the PFES product for much of this time. He has been responsible for many of Logica's projects to develop formulation applications based on PFES on behalf of various customers. He currently spends much of his time working on military expert systems for the UK Ministry of Defence. Paul has a BSc in Computer Studies from the University of East Anglia. He joined Logica on graduating in 1981.

Elizabeth A. Colbourn   Elizabeth Colbourn is Managing Director of Oxford Materials Ltd (UK), a position which she has held since September 1993. She is responsible for the development and promotion of software packages which can be used to design new materials and new processes. Previously, she established and led the materials modelling team at ICI plc, based at its Wilton Materials Research Centre in north-east England, where she carried out research on behalf of most of ICI's materials based businesses.

A Canadian by birth, she has been involved in materials modelling for both polymeric and inorganic systems for over 20 years, and is the author of over 50 publications in the scientific literature. She has a BSc in Chemistry from Queen's University at Kingston (Canada) and a DPhil in Theoretical Chemistry from the University of Oxford. She is a Chartered Chemist and a Fellow of the Royal Society of Chemistry, and is on the committee of the Molecular Modelling Group and Polar Solids Group of the RSC and of the Molecular Graphics and Modelling Society.

David Ganderton   David Ganderton studied at Brighton Technical College and the School of Pharmacy, University of London, UK and was awarded the degree of BPharm in 1958. He undertook postgraduate research in powder technology, receiving a PhD in 1962. Through teaching appointments at London, Sunderland and Glasgow, he specialised in industrial aspects of pharmacy. In 1970, he joined the Pharmaceuticals Division of ICI, now Zeneca Pharmaceuticals, in order to direct its research in drug delivery. Having progressed to the management of all aspects of analytical and product development, he left the company in 1985 to take the Chair of Pharmaceutics in the Department of Pharmacy, King's College London. He resigned from this post in 1990 but retains a teaching and research role as a visiting professor. He is presently the Technical Director of Co-ordinated Drug Development (CDD), an academic research group based at Bath University, where his specialty is pulmonary delivery of drugs.

Professor Ganderton is Chairman of the British Pharmacopoeia Commission and leads the UK Delegation to the European Pharmacopoeia. As a member of the latter's Expert Group 12, he has taken charge of the compendial control of products used in inhalation. He is a member of the Advisory Committee on NHS Drugs and the Chemistry, Pharmacy and Standards Sub-committee of the Committee of Safety of Medicines. For such services, an OBE was conferred in 1995.

Index